Vitamin C and the Common Cold

Vitamin C and the Common Cold

Linus Pauling

W. H. FREEMAN AND COMPANY
San Francisco

Printed in the United States of America

Library of Congress Catalog Card Number: 76-140232
ISBN: 0-7167-0159-6 (cloth); 0-7167-0160-X (paper)

65806

1 2 3 4 5 6 7 8 9

to
ALBERT SZENT-GYORGYI
who discovered ascorbic acid
and
IRWIN STONE
who aroused my interest in it

Contents

Vitamin C
and the
Common
Cold

Introduction

The idea that I should write this book developed gradually in my mind during the last five years. In April 1966 I received a letter from Dr. Irwin Stone, a biochemist whom I had met at the Carl Neuberg Medal Award dinner in New York the previous month. He mentioned in his letter that I had expressed a desire to live for the next fifteen or twenty years. He said that he would like to see me remain in good health for the next *fifty* years, and that he was accordingly sending me a description of his high-level ascorbic-acid* regimen, which he had developed during the preceding three decades. My wife

*In this book the terms "ascorbic acid" and "vitamin C" are used interchangeably (see Chapter 3).

and I began the regimen recommended by Dr. Stone. We noticed an increased feeling of wellbeing, and especially a striking decrease in the number of colds that we caught, and in their severity.

(Dr. Stone was, of course, exaggerating. I estimate that complete control of the common cold and associated disorders would increase the average life expectancy by two or three years. The improvement in the general state of health resulting from ingesting the optimum amount of ascorbic acid might lead to an equal additional increase in life expectancy.)

I gradually became aware of the existence of an extraordinary contradiction between the opinions of different people about the value of vitamin C in preventing and ameliorating the common cold. Many people believe that vitamin C helps prevent colds; on the other hand, most physicians deny that this vitamin has much value in treating the common cold. For example, in the discussion of the treatment of the common cold in his excellent book *Health* (1970) Dr. Benjamin A. Kogan makes the following statement: "Research has shown that vitamin C, in the form of fruit juice, however pleasant, is useless in preventing or shortening colds." Dr. John M. Adams does not mention vitamin C in his recent book *Viruses and Colds: the Modern Plague* (1967).

The difference of opinion was brought sharply to my attention by the publication of an article about vitamin C in the magazine *Mademoiselle* in November 1969. I was quoted as supporting the use of large amounts of vitamin C. Dr. Fredrick J. Stare, described as "one of the country's Big Names in nutrition," was quoted as saying "Vitamin C and colds—that was disproved twenty years ago. I'll tell you about just one very careful study. Of five thousand students at the University of Minnesota, half were given large doses of C, half a placebo.

Their medical histories were followed for two years—and no difference was found in the frequency, severity, or duration of their colds. And yes, stores of C are depleted in massive, lingering infection—not in week-long colds."

The study to which Dr. Stare was referring had been carried out by Cowan, Diehl, and Baker; the article describing their results was published in 1942 (see Chapter 5). When I read this article I found that the study involved only about four hundred students, rather than five thousand, that it was continued for half a year, not two years, and that it involved use of only 200 milligrams of vitamin C per day, which is not a large dose. Moreover, the investigators reported that the students receiving the vitamin C had 15 percent fewer colds than those receiving a placebo.

The fact that Dr. Stare, as well as the investigators themselves (Cowan, Diehl, and Baker), had not considered a decrease by 15 percent in the incidence of colds as important suggested to me that an examination of the medical literature might provide more information about this matter. The August 1967 issue of the journal *Nutrition Reviews* contained a brief editorial article about vitamin C and the common cold, in which a number of articles on the subject were mentioned. Dr. Stare, who is a professor in the Department of Nutrition of the School of Public Health of Harvard University, was editor of this journal at that time. The conclusion reported in this article was that "there is no conclusive evidence that ascorbic acid has any protective effect against, or any therapeutic effect on, the course of the common cold in healthy people not depleted of ascorbic acid. There is also no evidence for a general antiviral, or symptomatic prophylactic effect of ascorbic acid."

I examined the reports mentioned in this editorial article (they are all discussed in Chapter 5 and Appendix III), and found that my own conclusions, on the basis of the studies themselves, were different from those expressed in the editorial article.

We may ask why the physicians and authorities on nutrition have remained so lacking in enthusiasm about a substance that was reported three decades ago to decrease the incidence of colds by 15 percent, when taken regularly in rather small daily amounts. I surmise that several factors have contributed to this lack of enthusiasm. In the search for a drug to combat a disease the effort is usually made to find one that is 100 percent effective. (I must say that I do not understand, however, why Cowan, Diehl, and Baker did not repeat their study with use of larger amounts of vitamin C per day.) Also, there seems to have existed a feeling that the intake of vitamin C should be kept as small as possible, even though this vitamin is known to have extremely low toxicity. This attitude is, of course, proper for *drugs*—substances not normally present in the human body and almost always rather highly toxic—but it does not apply to ascorbic acid. Another factor has probably been the lack of interest of the drug companies in a natural substance that is available at a low price and cannot be patented.

Dr. Stone's letter to me came at a time in my own development when it was possible for me to contribute to the subject. For many years, since 1935, I had been working on the general problem of the relation between physiological activity and molecular structure of the substances present in the human body. With my students and colleagues I had worked on the structure of the complex molecules of hemoglobin and other proteins, on the nature of antibodies (which provide a natural protection against infectious disease), on the nature of sickle-cell anemia and other molecular diseases, and, beginning in 1954, on the possibility that mental diseases often have a molecular basis.

In the course of these investigations I became deeply interested in the vitamins, and I learned that Dr. A. Hoffer and Dr. H. Osmond had begun treating schizophrenic patients with large doses of a vitamin, either niacin or niacinamide. I was astonished to read that they recommended the use of between 3 grams and 18 grams of niacin or niacinamide per day in the treatment of schizophrenia. This amount is hundreds of times as much as is needed to prevent the dietary deficiency disease pellagra. I had formulated some ideas about why, for some people, at any rate, improved health might result from an increase in intake of certain vitamins, and later on, in 1968, I published these ideas (see Chapter 7). Dr. Stone's letter, together with some studies by other people, and those by my colleague Professor Arthur B. Robinson and me on ascorbic acid in relation to schizophrenia were significant in encouraging me to examine the matter of vitamin C and the common cold, as described in this book.

I hope that the arguments that are presented here will be found so convincing, by both the public and physicians, as to lead to the widespread use of ascorbic acid in increased amounts to control respiratory infections. I do not know how effective this regimen really is—whether 90 percent of all colds can be stopped, or perhaps only 75 percent or 50 percent. Even 25 percent success would be well worth while. Professor Robinson and I are now carrying on a rather small study to answer this question. I hope that other investigators in the field of public health will carry out some large-scale studies, and that the National Institutes of Health of the Department of Health, Education, and Welfare and other agencies will allocate large sums of money to support studies of this sort, as is justified by the importance of the common cold as a cause of discomfort and disability.

The common cold is an infection by viruses that circulate throughout the world. It rapidly dies out in a small isolated population. If the incidence of colds could be decreased enough throughout the world the common cold would disappear, as smallpox has in the British Isles. I foresee the achievement of this goal, perhaps within a decade or two, for some parts of the world. Some period of quarantine of travelers might be needed, so long as a major part of the world's people are poverty stricken and especially subject to infectious diseases because of malnutrition, including lack of ascorbic acid in the proper amount.

It will take decades to eradicate the common cold completely, but it can, I believe, be controlled almost entirely in the United States and some other countries within a few years, through improvement of the nutrition of the people by an adequate intake of ascorbic acid. I look forward to witnessing this step toward a better world.

The Common Cold

The common cold causes a tremendous amount of human suffering. The average incidence of colds is about three per person per year. A cold usually lasts from three to ten days. During part of this period the victim may feel miserable. If he is wise, he spends a few days in bed. The cold may be followed by serious complications—bronchitis, sinus infection, infection of the middle ear, infection of the mastoid bone (mastoiditis), meningitis, bronchopneumonia or lobar pneumonia, or exacerbation of some other disease, such as arthritis or kidney disease or heart disease.

The common cold (acute coryza) is an inflammation of the upper respiratory tract caused by infection with a virus.* This infection alters the physiology of the mucous membrane of the nose, the paranasal sinuses, and the throat. The common cold occurs more often than all other diseases combined. The common cold does not occur in small isolated communities. Exposure to the virus, carried by other persons, is needed. For example, the Norwegian island of Spitsbergen used to be isolated during seven months of the year. The 507 residents of the principal town of the island, Longyear, were nearly free of colds through the cold winter, with only four colds recorded in three months. Then within two weeks after the arrival of the first ship some two hundred of the residents had become ill with colds (Paul and Freese, 1933).

Development of a cold after exposure to the virus is determined to some extent by the state of health of the person and by environmental factors. Fatigue, chilling of the body, wearing of wet clothing and wet shoes, and the presence of irritating substances in the air make it more likely that the cold will develop. Experimental studies indicate, however, that these factors, fatigue, chilling, wearing of wet clothing, and presence of irritating substances in the air, are not so important as is generally believed (Andrewes, 1965; Debré and Celers, 1970, page 539). The period of incubation, between exposure and the manifestation of symptoms, is usually two or three days. The first symptoms are a feeling of roughness or soreness of the throat, development of a nasal discharge, attacks of sneezing, and a sensation of fullness and irritation in the upper

---

*A discussion of the many viruses that can cause the common cold is given in the book *The Common Cold*, by Sir Christopher Andrewes, 1965. (Note that full bibliographic information is given for all references, listed alphabetically by name of the first author, beginning on page 111.)

respiratory tract. Headache, general malaise (an indefinite feeling of uneasiness or discomfort), and chills (a sensation of coldness attended with convulsive shaking of the body, pinched face, pale skin, and blue lips) are often present. A slight increase in temperature, usually to not over 101°F (38.3°C), may occur. The mucous membranes of the nose and pharynx are swollen. One nostril or both nostrils may be blocked by the thickened secretions. The skin around the nostrils may become sore, and cold sores (caused by the virus *Herpes simplex*) may develop on the lips.

The customary treatment for the common cold includes resting in bed, drinking fruit juice or water, ingesting a simple and nutritious diet, preventing irritants such as tobacco smoke from entering the respiratory tract, and alleviating the symptoms to some extent by the use of aspirin, phenacetin, antihistamines, and other drugs (see Chapter 9). After some days the tissues of the nose and throat, weakened by the virus infection, often are invaded by bacteria. This secondary infection may cause the nasal secretions to become purulent (to contain pus). Also, the secondary infection may spread to the sinuses, the middle ears, the tonsils, the pharynx, the larynx, the trachea, the bronchi, and the lungs. As mentioned above, mastoiditis, meningitis, and other serious infections may follow. Control of the common cold thus would lead to a decrease in the incidence of more serious diseases.

Not everyone is susceptible to infection with the common cold. Most investigators have noted that an appreciable proportion of the population, 6 to 10 percent, never have colds. This fact provides justification for hope that a significant decrease in the number of colds can be achieved through increase in the resistance of individuals to viral infection. It is likely that the ability of 6 to 10 percent of the population to avoid colds is the result of their natural powers of resistance. Like other physiological properties, the resistance of individuals to viral infection probably can be represented by a distribution curve that has approximately the normal bell shape. The 6 to 10 percent of the population that are resistant to colds presumably correspond to the tail end of the curve, those people with the largest natural powers of resisting viral infections. If in some way the natural resistance of the whole population could be shifted upward, a larger percentage of the population would lie in the range corresponding to complete resistance to the infection, and would never have colds. This argument indicates strongly that a study of the factors involved in the natural resistance to viral infection, such as nutritional factors, could lead to a significant decrease in the susceptibility of the population as a whole to the common cold. (See, for example, Debré and Celers, 1970, page 539.)

I have made a rough estimate of the significance of the common cold, measured in dollars. Let us assume that the average loss of time because of serious illness with the common cold is seven days per person per year. The person suffering from a cold or series of colds during the year might stay away from work, or he might have a decreased effectiveness, or might be sufficiently ill to feel that the seven days are wasted. In any case, a measure of the damage done by the common cold might be roughly taken as his loss of productivity and income for the seven days during the year when he is most seriously ill. The personal income of the people of the United States is about eight hundred billion dollars per year. The income per week is this quantity divided by 52, which is about fifteen billion dollars. We may accordingly be justified in saying that the damage done by the common cold to the people of the

United States each year can be described roughly as corresponding to a monetary loss of fifteen billion dollars per year.*

This estimate corresponds to a loss in income or its equivalent in wellbeing of about seventy-five dollars per year per person in the United States.

It is easy to understand why the people of the United States spend hundreds of millions of dollars per year on cold medicines, despite their limited effectiveness, in an effort to reduce their physical discomfort and loss of income.

In the medical literature it is usually said that no clearly effective method of treatment of the common cold has been developed. The various drugs that are prescribed or recommended may have some value in making the patient more comfortable, by giving him relief from some of the more distressing symptoms, but they have little effect on the duration of the cold. I believe, on the other hand, that most colds can be prevented or largely ameliorated by control of the diet, without the use of any drugs. The dietary substance that is involved is vitamin C, which is known to be the substance ascorbic acid.**

Ascorbic acid is a food. It is, in fact, an essential food for all human beings. It is present, in greater or smaller amounts, in many ordinary foodstuffs, including fruits, vegetables, and meats. For about forty years it has been available in pure form, either separated from a fruit or vegetable in which it occurs

---

*A somewhat smaller estimate, five billion dollars per year, was given by Fabricant and Conklin in their book *The Dangerous Cold*, 1965.

**As noted in the Introduction, the words "ascorbic acid" and "vitamin C" are used interchangeably. I have retained use of the term "vitamin C" in order to emphasize the role of ascorbic acid as an essential nutrient, "ascorbic acid" to call attention to its existence as a pure substance.

or made from a sugar (glucose or sorbose) by a simple chemical reaction, similar to the chemical reactions that take place continually in living plants and animals.

A person's health depends in part on the foods that he eats. Certain amounts of some foods are needed for life. These essential foods include the essential amino acids, essential fats, certain minerals, and the various vitamins, including vitamin C.

A person who eats no vitamin C, even though his diet is adequate in other respects, will become sick, and then die, in a few months. A small intake of vitamin C, which for many people may lie somewhere within the limits 5 mg (milligrams) to 15 mg per day, is enough to prevent a human being from dying of vitamin C deficiency, which is called scurvy. The amount that keeps him from dying of scurvy may not, however, be the amount that puts him in the best of health. The amount that puts him in the best of health, which may be called the optimum amount, is not reliably known; but there is some evidence that for different people it lies in the range between 250 mg and 10,000 mg per day; that is, between 1/4 g (gram) and 10 g per day.*

The evidence indicating the need for these larger amounts of vitamin C in order to achieve the best of health, including protection against the common cold, is presented in later chapters in this book. The discussion of the optimum intake of vitamin C for averting and ameliorating the common cold is given in Chapters 5 and 10.

The relatively low cost of dietary control of the common cold, in comparison with the monetary equivalent of the damage

---

*One pound equals 453.6 g, and one ounce equals 28.35 g. One kilogram equals 2.2 pounds. A level teaspoonful of ascorbic acid is 4.4 g.

done by the disease and the large amounts of money now spent on ineffective medicines, is discussed in Chapter 10.

It is, of course, essential that everyone consult his physician in case of serious illness. An improved diet should improve your general health; but you cannot hope that it will protect you completely from "the rotten diseases of the south, the guts-griping, ruptures, catarrhs, loads o' gravel i' the back, lethargies, cold palsies, raw eyes, dirt-rotten livers, wheezing lungs, bladders full of imposthume, sciaticas, limekilns i' the palm, incurable boneache, and the riveled fee-simple of the tetter" (Shakespeare, *Troilus and Cressida*).

CHAPTER 2

Scurvy

Scurvy is a deficiency disease. It is caused by a deficiency of a certain food, vitamin C, in the diet. People who receive no vitamin C become sick and die.

Scurvy has been known for hundreds of years, but it was not until 1911 that its cause was clearly recognized to be a dietary deficiency. Until about a century ago the disease was very common among sailors on board ships taking long voyages. It also frequently broke out among soldiers in an army on campaign, in communities in times of scarcity of food, in cities under siege, and in prisons and workhouses. Scurvy plagued the California gold miners 120 years ago, and the Alaskan gold miners 70 years ago.

The onset of scurvy is marked by a failure of strength, including restlessness and rapid exhaustion on making effort. The skin becomes sallow or dusky. The patient complains of pains in the muscles. He is mentally depressed. Later, his face looks haggard. His gums ulcerate, his teeth drop out, and his breath is fetid. Hemorrhages of large size penetrate the muscles and other tissues, giving him the appearance of being extensively bruised. The later stages of the disease are marked by profound exhaustion, diarrhea, and pulmonary and kidney troubles, leading to death.

The ravages of scurvy among the early sea voyagers were terrible. On a long voyage the sailors lived largely on biscuits, salt beef, and salt pork, which contain very little vitamin C. Between 9 July 1497 and 20 May 1498 the Portuguese navigator Vasco da Gama made the voyage of discovery of the searoute around Africa to India, sailing from Lisbon to Calicut. During this voyage one hundred of his crew of 160 died of scurvy. In the year 1577 a Spanish galleon was found adrift in the Sargasso Sea, with everyone on board dead of scurvy. Late in 1740 the British Admiral George Anson set out with a squadron of six ships manned by 961 sailors. By June 1741, when he reached the island of Juan Fernandez, the number of sailors had decreased to 335, more than half of his men having died of scurvy.

The idea that scurvy could be prevented by a proper diet developed only slowly. In 1536 the French explorer Jacques Cartier discovered the St. Lawrence River, and sailed up the river to the site of the present city of Quebec, where Cartier and his men spent the winter. Twenty-five of the men died of scurvy, and many others were very sick. A friendly Indian advised them to make a tea with use of the leaves and bark of the arbor vitae tree, *Thuja occidentalis*. The treatment was beneficial. The leaves or needles of this tree have now been shown to contain about 50 mg of vitamin C per 100 g.

In 1747, while in the British naval service, the Scottish physician James Lind carried out a now famous experiment with twelve patients severely ill with scurvy. He placed them all on the same diet, except for one item, one of the reputed remedies that he was testing. To each of two patients he gave two oranges and one lemon per day; to two others, cider; to the others, dilute sulfuric acid, or vinegar, or sea water, or a mixture of drugs. At the end of six days the two who had received the citrus fruits were well, while the other ten remained ill. Lind carried out further studies, which he later described in his book, *A Treatise on Scurvy*, which was published in 1753.

There followed a period of controversy about the value of the juice of citrus fruits in preventing scurvy. Some of the unsuccessful trials involved the use of orange, lemon, and lime juice that had been boiled down to a syrup. We know now that most of the ascorbic acid in the juice was destroyed by this process. Finally, however, in 1795, forty-eight years after Lind had carried out his striking experiment, the British Admiralty ordered that a daily ration of lime juice* (not boiled to a syrup) be given to the sailors, and scurvy disappeared from the British Navy.

The spirit of free enterprise remained dominant in the British Board of Trade, however, and scurvy continued to ravage the British merchant marine for seventy years longer. In 1865 the Board of Trade finally passed a similar lime-juice regulation for the merchant marine.

---

*Hence the name Lime-juicer or Limey for an English sailor.

The striking story of the experience of the great English explorer Captain James Cook in the control of scurvy among his crews on his Pacific voyages during the period 1768 to 1780 has been told by Kodicek and Young in the *Notes and Records of the Royal Society of London* (1969). These authors quote the following song by the sailor T. Perry, a member of the crew of Captain Cook's flagship H.M.S. Resolution:

> We were all hearty seamen, no colds did we fear
> And we have from all sickness entirely kept clear
> Thanks be to the Captain, he has proved so good
> Amongst all the Islands to give us fresh food.

This song, written two hundred years ago, indicates that Cook's sailors believed that fresh food (containing vitamin C) provided them with protection against colds, as well as against other diseases.

Captain Cook made use of many antiscorbutic agents. Whenever the ships reached shore he ordered the sailors to gather fruits, vegetables, berries, and green plants. In South America, Australia, and Alaska the leaves of spruce trees were gathered and made into an infusion called spruce beer. Nettletops and wild leeks were boiled with wheat and served at breakfast. Cook began one voyage with a supply of 7860 pounds of sauerkraut, enough to provide two pounds per week for a period of a year for each of the seventy men on board his first flagship, the Endeavour. (Sauerkraut contains a good amount of vitamin C, about 30 mg per 100 g.) The results of his care was that, despite some illness, not a single member of his crew died of scurvy during his three Pacific voyages, carried out at a time when scurvy was still ravaging the crews of most vessels on such protracted voyages.

The English admiral Sir John Hawkins (1532-1595) knew that the juice of citrus fruits is effective in preventing scurvy:

> It was found on a very long voyage that the crew suffered from scurvy in proportion to the length of time they were restricted to dry foods, and that they recovered rapidly as soon as they got access to a supply of succulent plants. This requisite for health is obviously the most difficult of all things to procure aboard ship, and efforts were made to find a substitute capable of marine transport. From the time of Hawkins (1593) downwards the opinion has been expressed by all the most intelligent travelers that a substitute is to be found in the juice of fruits of the orange tribes, such as oranges, lemons, etc. But in its natural state this is expensive and troublesome to carry, so that skippers and owners for a couple of centuries found it expedient to be skeptical. The pictures of scurvy as it appeared during the 18th century are horrible in the extreme. (In the article "Dietetics," *Encyclopedia Britannica*, 9th Edition, Volume 7, 1878.)

At the present time scurvy, complicated by other deficiency diseases, is found in populations that are ravaged by starvation and severe malnutrition, usually as a result of poverty. In the United States scurvy is also occasionally observed in people who are not poverty-stricken: among infants 6 to 18 months old who are fed a formula without vitamin supplement, and such persons as middle-aged or elderly bachelors or widowers who for convenience ingest an unsatisfactory diet, deficient in the essential nutrients.

CHAPTER 3

The Discovery
of Vitamins

In the article on scurvy in the Eleventh Edition of the En-
cyclopedia Britannica (1911) the statement is made that the
incidence of scurvy depends upon the nature of the food, and
that it is disputed whether the cause is the *absence* of certain
constituents in the food, or the *presence* of some actual poison.

The study of another disease, beriberi, was then in a similar
state. Beriberi was prevalent in eastern Asia, where rice is
the staple food, and was found also in the Pacific islands and
South America. The disease involves paralysis and numbness,
starting from the legs and leading to cardiac and respiratory
disorders and to death. In the Dutch East Indies, about one
hundred years ago, soldiers, sailors, prisoners, mine workers

and plantation workers, and persons admitted to a hospital for treatment of minor ailments were dying of the disease by the thousands. Young men in seemingly good health sometimes died suddenly, in terrible distress through inability to breathe. In 1886 a young Dutch physician, Christiaan Eijkman, was asked by the Dutch government to study the disease. For three years he made little progress. Then he noticed that the chickens in the laboratory chickenhouse were dying of a paralytic disease closely resembling beriberi. His studies of the chickens' disease were suddenly brought to an end, when the chickens that had not yet died recovered and no new cases developed. He found on investigating the circumstances that the man in charge of the chickens had been feeding them, from 17 June to 27 November, on polished rice (with the husks removed) prepared in the military hospital kitchen for the hospital patients. Then a new cook took charge of the kitchen; he refused to "allow military rice to be taken for civilian chickens."* The disease had broken out among the chickens on 10 July and disappeared during the last days of November.

It was immediately confirmed that a diet of polished rice causes death of chickens in three or four weeks, whereas they remain in good health when fed unpolished rice. A study of 300,000 prisoners in 101 prisons in the Dutch East Indies was then made, and it was found that the incidence of beriberi was three hundred times as great in the prisons where polished rice was used as a staple diet as in those where unpolished rice was used.

---

*These are the words used by Eijkman in his Nobel address, when he received half of the Nobel Prize for Physiology and Medicine, 1929, allotted to him for his discovery of vitamin B_1, deficiency of which is the cause of beriberi.

Eijkman found that he could isolate an extract from the bran of the rice that had protective power against beriberi. At first he thought that some substance in the bran acted as an antidote for a toxin assumed to be present in polished rice, but by 1907 he and his collaborator Grijns had concluded that the bran contains a nutrient substance that is required for good health.

In the meantime a number of investigators had been studying the nutritional value of foods. It was shown that for good health certain minerals are needed (compounds of sodium, potassium, iron, copper, and other metals), as well as proteins, carbohydrates, and fats. The Swiss biochemist Lunin found, in 1881, that mice died when they were fed a mixture of purified protein, carbohydrate, fat, and minerals, whereas those fed the same diet with the addition of some milk survived. He concluded that "a natural food such as milk must therefore contain besides these known principal ingredients small quantities of unknown substances essential to life." Similar observations were made in the same laboratory (in Basel) ten years later by another Swiss biochemist, Socin, who found that small amounts of either egg yolk or milk, in addition to the purified diet, sufficed to keep the mice in good health. In 1905 the Dutch physiologist Pekelharing found that very small amounts of the unknown essential substances in milk were enough to keep the animals in good health. Between 1905 and 1912 the English biochemist F. Gowland Hopkins carried on similar studies with rats, showing that, in addition to purified protein, carbohydrate, fat, and minerals, a small amount of milk is needed to keep the rats in good health. His results were announced in 1911 and published in detail in 1912. Hopkins shared the 1929 Nobel Prize for Physiology and Medicine with Eijkman.

In 1911 Casimir Funk, a Polish biochemist then working in the Lister Institute in London, published his theory of "vitamines," based upon his review of the existing knowledge about diseases associated with faulty nutrition. He suggested that four such substances are present in natural foods, and that they serve to provide protection against four diseases, beriberi, scurvy, pellagra, and rickets. Funk coined the word vitamine from the Latin word *vita*, life, and the chemical term amine, a member of a class of compounds of nitrogen. Later, when it was found that some of these essential substances do not contain nitrogen, the word was changed to vitamin.

During the following years a number of efforts were made to separate pure vitamin C from lemon juice and other foods. The pure vitamin was finally obtained, in 1928, by a scientist, Albert Szent-Györgyi, who was working on another problem, and at first did not know that his new substance was vitamin C. He named the substance hexuronic acid, and later changed the name to ascorbic acid. Szent-Györgyi was given the Nobel Prize for Physiology and Medicine for the year 1937, in recognition of his discoveries concerning the biological oxidation processes, with especial reference to vitamin C and to the role of fumaric acid in these processes.

Albert Szent-Györgyi was born in Budapest on 16 September 1893. He studied medicine in Budapest, and immediately began his career as an investigator in the fields of physiology and biochemistry. While he was working in the Netherlands in 1922 he began a study of the oxidation reactions that cause a brown pigmentation to appear in certain fruits as they decay. In the course of these studies he found that cabbages contain a reducing agent (an agent that can combine with oxygen), and that the adrenal glands of animals contain the same reducing agent, or a similar one. Because of his interest in physiological oxidation-reduction reactions he began to try to isolate this reducing agent from the plant tissues and from adrenal glands. In 1927 he received a fellowship from the Rockefeller Foundation, permitting him to spend a year in the laboratory of F. Gowland Hopkins in Cambridge, England. Here he succeeded in isolating the substance from plant tissues and from the adrenal glands of animals. He then spent a year in the Mayo Foundation, Rochester, Minnesota, where he succeeded in obtaining 25 grams of the substance, hexuronic acid. In 1930 he returned to Hungary, where he found that Hungarian paprika contains large amounts of the substance. He and his collaborators, and also the American investigators Waugh and King, showed in 1932 that Szent-Györgyi's substance was vitamin C. Szent-Györgyi himself had found that the chemical formula of the substance is $C_6H_8O_6$. He gave some of the crystalline material to the English sugar chemist W. M. Haworth, who determined its structural formula.

Within a short time the value of ascorbic acid in improving health began to be recognized. The pure substance soon became available in drug stores and food stores. For many years, however, there was an astounding lack of interest by physicians in the use of this important food for the benefit of their patients. I believe that soon the attitude of physicians toward ascorbic acid and other important nutrients will undergo a significant change.

The Properties of Ascorbic Acid

Ascorbic acid is an essential food for human beings. As noted earlier, an intake of about 10 mg per day is enough to provide protection against scurvy for most people, but to achieve the best health a much larger intake is probably needed.

The optimum intake of ascorbic acid—that is, the daily amount of this food that leads to the best of health—is not known, and no doubt it varies from person to person. It is my opinion that for most people the optimum daily intake is somewhere between 250 mg and 10 g.

These amounts are much larger than the daily dietary allowance recommended in 1968 by the Food and Nutrition Board of the National Research Council. The recommendation of this

Board, said to be designed for the maintenance of good nutrition of practically all healthy people in the United States, is 35 mg per day for infants, 40 mg per day for children, increasing to 55 mg per day for women and 60 mg per day for men. In making its recommendation the Board stated that the minimal daily intake of ascorbic acid needed to prevent scurvy is about 10 mg, and that the somewhat larger amounts recommended should provide a generous increment for individual variability and a surplus to compensate for potential losses in food. The idea that beneficial effects would result from a larger intake of ascorbic acid was rejected, on the basis of reports that improvement in physical and psychomotor performances of men had not been improved by supplements of between 70 mg and 300 mg of ascorbic acid per day, and that the occurrence of bleeding gums in military personnel was not affected by supplements of 100 mg or 200 mg per day for periods of three weeks. There are, however, many published reports about beneficial effects of ascorbic acid ingested in larger amounts. Some of these reports are discussed later in this chapter and, with respect to the common cold and other infections, in the following chapter and Appendix III.

Ascorbic acid is not a dangerous substance. It is described in the medical literature as "virtually nontoxic." Guinea pigs that were given one half of one percent of their body weight of ascorbic acid per day for a period of days showed no symptoms of toxicity. Human beings are reported to have eaten 40 g per day for a month (Stone, 1967) and as much as 100 g per day for a few days (Herjanic and Moss-Herjanic, 1967) with no symptoms of toxicity. A large amount (several grams) of ascorbic acid eaten without other food may cause an upset stomach and diarrhea in some people (hence the recommendation in Chapter 10 that it usually be taken at the end of a meal), but more serious side effects have not been reported.

Ascorbic acid may be described as no more toxic than ordinary sugar (sucrose), and far less toxic than ordinary salt (sodium chloride). There is no reported case of the death of any person from eating too much ascorbic acid, nor, indeed, of serious illness from this cause.

Ascorbic acid is a white, crystalline powder, with large solubility in water. Its solution has an acidic taste, resembling that of orange juice.

Ordinary ascorbic acid is also called L-ascorbic acid. There is another substance, D-ascorbic acid, that is closely related to L-ascorbic acid; the two substances contain the same atoms, bonded together in essentially the same way, but with a spatial relationship corresponding to reflection in a mirror. The letters D and L indicate righthanded (dextro) and lefthanded (levo). Only L-ascorbic acid has vitamin-C activity. The name ascorbic acid without a prefix is used only in referring to L-ascorbic acid, vitamin C itself.

Ascorbic acid is found in many foodstuffs. Large amounts, 100 mg to 350 mg per 100 g (that is, between 0.10 and 0.35 percent of the weight of the food) are contained in green peppers, red peppers, parsley, and turnip greens. Orange juice, lemon juice, lime juice, grapefruit juice, tomato juice, mustard greens, spinach, and brussels sprouts contain a good quantity of ascorbic acid, from 25 mg to 100 mg per 100 g. Green peas and green beans, sweet corn, asparagus, pineapple, tomatoes, gooseberries, cranberries, cucumbers, and lettuce contain from 10 mg to 25 mg per 100 g. Somewhat smaller amounts, less than 10 mg per 100 g, are found in eggs, milk, carrots, beets, and cooked meat.

The ascorbic acid in foodstuffs is easily destroyed by cooking at high temperatures, especially in the presence of copper, iron, and other metals. Cooked foods usually retain only about half of the ascorbic acid present in the raw foods. The loss of the vitamin can be kept to a minimum by cooking for a short period of time, with a minimum amount of water, and with the water not discarded, because it has extracted some of the vitamin from the food.

A good ordinary diet, including green vegetables and orange or tomato juice, may provide 100 mg to 300 mg of ascorbic acid per day. To obtain larger amounts of this important food the pure substance, crystalline ascorbic acid, may be ingested.

Pure ascorbic acid (Ascorbic Acid U.S.P., L-Ascorbic Acid, Vitamin C) is available in some drug stores and food stores as a powder, fine crystals, or coarse crystals, and also, with a binder or filler added, as tablets. This ascorbic acid is some-times described as synthetic ascorbic acid. It is identical with the ascorbic acid present in natural foodstuffs, and it is, in fact, usually made from a natural sugar by a process involving two chemical reactions. The usual starting material is dextrose, which is also called glucose, grape sugar, honey sugar, corn sugar, or starch sugar. It is present in honey and other natural foods. Its chemical formula is $C_6H_{12}O_6$. It is converted into L-ascorbic acid, $C_6H_8O_6$, by oxidation reactions which remove four hydrogen atoms to form two molecules of water.

Many animals are able to manufacture their own ascorbic acid; they do not require ascorbic acid (vitamin C) as an essential food, and they never suffer from scurvy. These animals manufacture the ascorbic acid in their bodies (in the liver or the kidney) from dextrose by essentially the same reactions that are used to make ascorbic acid in the laboratory and on a commercial scale.

Ascorbic acid in the human body and in other animals seems to have many functions. These functions have been studied in the guinea pig and the monkey, both of which, like human beings, require ascorbic acid in their food, as a vitamin. It has been found that an insufficient supply of this essential food causes the animal to show symptoms of scurvy, including intramuscular and subcutaneous hemorrhages, tenderness of joints, a general weakening of connective tissue (skin, tendons, walls of blood vessels), lethargy, loss of appetite, and anemia. Ascorbic acid is needed for the healing of wounds, including burns. With a low intake of ascorbic acid wounds heal only slowly and the scar tissue is weak, so that the wounds break open again easily. Increase in the intake of ascorbic acid leads to rapid healing and to the formation of strong scar tissue (see Figure 1, on the next page).

It has been found that a large intake of ascorbic acid increases the capacity of resistance of the guinea pig, the rat, and the monkey to a cold environment (Dugal, 1961). In human beings, a fall in the concentration of ascorbic acid in the blood has been observed to follow exposure to the stress of surgery, accidental wounds, and burns, indicating the need for a larger supply of the vitamin. Ascorbic acid in increased amounts has been used in the treatment of burns, injuries, infections, rheumatic disease, and allergies (Holmes, 1946; Yandell, 1951).

In 1964 Dr. James Greenwood, Jr., clinical professor of neurosurgery in Baylor University College of Medicine, reported his observations on the effect of an increased intake of ascorbic acid in preserving the integrity of intervertebral discs and preventing back trouble. He recommended the use of 500 mg per day with an increase to 1000 mg per day if there were any discomfort or if work or strenuous exercise were anticipated. He said that evidence from most patients

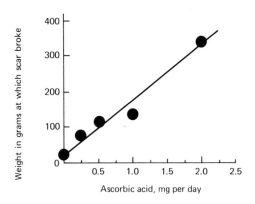

FIGURE 1

Strength of scar tissue in guinea-pig skin in dependence on the amount of ascorbic acid in the diet (0, 0.25, 0.5, 1, and 2 mg per day). The scars had been formed during a 7-day period after the cuts, 1/4-inch long, had been made. It is seen that the scar tissue is four times as strong for an intake of 2 mg per day as for 0.25 mg per day (Bourne, 1946). Similar results for human beings have been reported by Wolfer, Farmer, Carroll, and Manshardt (1947)

indicated that muscular soreness experienced with exercise had been greatly reduced by these doses of ascorbic acid, but increased again when the vitamin was not taken. He concluded, from observation of over 500 cases, that "it can be stated with reasonable assurance that a significant percentage of patients with early disc lesions were able to avoid surgery by the use of large doses of vitamin C. Many of these patients after a few months or years stopped their vitamin C and symptoms recurred. When they were placed back on the vitamin the symptoms disappeared. Some, of course, eventually came to surgery."

It has also been reported that the cancers that often appear in the bladders of cigar smokers and other users of tobacco regress if the patient ingests a sufficient amount of ascorbic acid, 1 g per day or more. Schlegel, Pipkin, Nishimura, and Schultz (1970) found the ascorbic-acid level of the urine to be about half as great for smokers as for nonsmokers, and to be low for patients with bladder tumors. They also found with mice that implantation in the bladder of a pellet containing 3-hydroxyanthranilic acid (a derivative of the amino acid tryptophan) caused bladder tumors to develop if the mice were receiving a normal diet, but not if they had extra ascorbic acid in their drinking water. The authors suggest that the ascorbic acid prevents the oxidation of 3-hydroxyanthranilic acid to a cancerogenic oxidation product. They state that "there seems to be reason to consider the beneficial effects of an adequate ascorbic acid level in the urine (corresponding to a rate of intake of 1.5 g per day) as a possible preventive measure in regard to bladder tumor formation and recurrence." They also call attention to investigations indicating that ascorbic acid may have a beneficial effect on the aging process of atherosclerosis, the hardening and thickening of the walls of the arteries (Willis and Fishman, 1955; Sokoloff and others, 1966).

Patients with various infectious diseases have been reported to benefit from treatment with ascorbic acid. Baetgen in 1961 reported the successful treatment of epidemic hepatitis in 245 children with use of 10 g of ascorbic acid per day. Several investigators, most recently Hindson (1968), have reported that prickly heat is cured by the ingestion of 0.5 to 1 g per day.

An interesting investigation of the relation between intelligence, as indicated by the results of standard mental ability tests, and the concentration of ascorbic acid in the blood plasma has been reported by Kubala and Katz (1960). The subjects were 351 students in four schools (kindergarten to college) in three cities. They were initially divided into the higher-ascorbic-acid group (with more than 1.10 mg of ascorbic acid per 100 ml of blood plasma) and the lower-ascorbic-acid group (less than 1.10 mg per 100 ml) on the basis of analysis of blood samples. By matching pairs on a socio-economic basis (family income, education of father and mother), 72 subjects in the higher-ascorbic-acid group and 72 in the lower-ascorbic-acid group were selected. It was found that the average intelligence quotient of the higher-ascorbic-acid group was greater than that of the lower-ascorbic-acid group in each of the four schools; for all 72 pairs of subjects the average IQ values were 113.22 and 108.71, respectively, with an average difference 4.51. The probability that a difference this great would be found in a similar test on a uniform population is less than 5 percent; hence the observed difference in average IQ of the two groups is statistically significant.

The subjects in both groups were then given supplementary orange juice during a period of six months, and the tests were repeated. The average intelligence quotient for those in the initially higher-ascorbic-acid group had increased very little (by only 0.02), whereas that for the lower group had increased by 3.54 IQ units. This difference in increase is also statistically significant (probability in a uniform population less than 5 percent.

The study was continued through a second school year with 32 pairs (64 subjects), with similar results. The relation between the average intelligence quotient and the average blood-plasma ascorbic-acid concentration for these 64 subjects tested four times during a period of 18 months is shown in Figure 2. These results indicate that the intelligence quotient is raised by 3.6 IQ units when the blood-plasma ascorbic-acid concentration is increased by 50 percent (from 1.03 to 1.55 mg per 100 ml). This increase would for many people result from

increasing the intake of ascorbic acid for an adult by 50 mg
per day (from 100 mg to 150 mg per day).

Kubala and Katz conclude that some of the variance in
intelligence-test performance is determined by the "temporary
nutritional state of the individual, at least with regards to citrus
or other products providing ascorbic acid." They suggest that
"alertness" or "sharpness" is diminished by a decreased intake
of ascorbic acid.

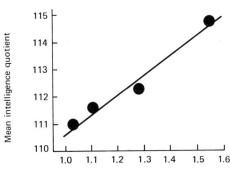

FIGURE 2

Relation between mean intelligence quotient (average IQ) and
mean concentration of ascorbic acid in the blood plasma for 64
school children. Four tests were made of each child, over a period
of 18 months. The plasma ascorbic-acid concentration was
changed by giving all the subjects extra orange juice during certain months. (Redrawn from Figure 1 of Kubala and Katz, 1960).

There is no indication in Figure 2 that maximum mental
ability has been reached at the value 1.55 mg of ascorbic acid
per 100 ml of blood plasma. This concentration corresponds
for a 70-kg (154-pound) adult to the daily ingestion of 180
mg of ascorbic acid. I conclude that for maximum mental per-

formance the daily allowance of ascorbic acid should be at
least three times the 60 mg recommended by the Food and
Nutrition Board of the U.S. National Research Council, and
at least nine times the 20 mg recommended by the corresponding British authority.

The ways in which ascorbic acid functions in the human
body are not well understood. It is a strong reducing agent,
and is readily converted into dehydroascorbic acid, $C_6H_6O_6$,
by oxidizing agents:

Ascorbic acid   Dehydroascorbic acid

This reaction is reversible (dehydroascorbic acid is easily reduced to ascorbic acid), and it is likely that the reducing power
of ascorbic acid and the oxidizing power of dehydroascorbic
acid are responsible for some of the physiological properties
of the substance.

Many of the results of deprivation of ascorbic acid, mentioned above, involve a deficiency in connective tissue. Connective tissue is largely responsible for the strength of bones, teeth,
skin, tendons, blood-vessel walls, and other parts of the body.
It consists mainly of the fibrous protein collagen. There is no
doubt that ascorbic acid is required for the synthesis of collagen

in the bodies of human beings and other animals. Collagen differs from other fibrous proteins in having a rather large content of the amino acid hydroxyproline. There is evidence that ascorbic acid is required for the conversion of proline into hydroxyproline. This is an oxidation reaction, and there is evidence also that ascorbic acid is involved in some other oxidation reactions in the tissues.

In his book *The Advancing Front of Medicine* (1941) an able science writer, George W. Gray, who was associated with the Rockefeller Foundation, wrote the following statement about ascorbic acid:

> Recent studies show that vitamin C is essential to the formation of the colloidal substance which serves as a pliable cement to bind tissue cells together. In healthy tissue, this binding material shows under the microscope as a clear jelly streaked with darker bands of firmer texture, like the reinforcing strips of steel in concrete. But in the absence of sufficient vitamin C, the bands do not form, the intercellular substance becomes more liquid, less binding, and the cells show a tendency to separate. The hemorrhages which accompany scurvy are consequences of this weakness in the intercellular substance. The cells forming the walls of small blood vessels separate, and through the gaps the blood leaks out. Microscopic studies show that as soon as vitamin C is administered to a scurvy patient, the bands reappear in the intercellular substance, and the separated cells once more join into continuous tissue.

Part of the mechanism of protection against disease is the destruction of bacteria by certain white cells in the blood, the phagocytes. In order to be effective in this way, the phagocytes must have a certain concentration of ascorbic acid in them. This fact provides a partial explanation of the effectiveness of ascorbic acid in providing protection against bacterial infections. The mechanism of its effectiveness against viral infections, such as the common cold, is not yet known. I have, however, formulated the hypothesis (which has not yet been tested by experiment) that the effectiveness of ascorbic acid in providing protection against virus diseases results from its function in the synthesis and activity of interferon in preventing the entry of virus particles into the cells. The discovery of interferon was reported in 1957 by Isaacs and Lindenmann. It is a protein that is produced by cells infected by a virus and that has the property of spreading to neighboring cells and changing them in such a way as to enable them to resist infection. In this way the interferon ameliorates the disease. I am sure that it will not be long before this hypothesis about the way in which ascorbic acid provides protection against virus diseases will be verified by experiment, or disproved by discovery of the actual mechanism. In the meantime we may make use of ascorbic acid for improving health in the ways indicated by experience, even though a detailed understanding of the mechanisms of its action has not yet been obtained.

CHAPTER 5

Ascorbic Acid and the Common Cold

I mentioned in the Introduction my decision to try to resolve the apparent contradiction between the opinions expressed by authorities in nutrition and my own experience, which supported the widely held belief that ascorbic acid has value in decreasing the incidence of infection and ameliorating the severity of the common cold.

The solution to the puzzle is a simple one. Ascorbic acid has only rather small value in providing protection against the common cold when it is taken in small amounts, but it has great value when it is taken in large amounts. As is explained below, the amount of protection increases with increase in the amount of ingested ascorbic acid, and becomes nearly complete with 4 g to 10 g per day taken at the immediate onset of the cold, as recommended by Dr. Irwin Stone and Dr. Edmé Régnier.

Most of the studies referred to in the editorial article in the August 1967 issue of *Nutrition Reviews* involved giving small amounts of ascorbic acid to the subjects, usually 200 mg per day. These studies indicate that such small amounts of ascorbic acid have some protective value, not very great, against the common cold.

In carrying out such a test, the best experiments are those in which the subjects are divided into two groups, in a random way, with the substance being tested (ascorbic acid) administered to the subjects in one group, and a placebo (an inactive material resembling the preparation to be tested: for example, a capsule containing citric acid might be used as a placebo for ascorbic acid) administered to those of the other group. In a blind experiment the subjects do not know whether or not they are receiving the placebo. Sometimes a double-blind study is made, in which the investigators evaluating the effects of the preparation and the placebo do not know which of the subjects received the preparation and which received the placebo until the study is completed, this information being kept by some other person.

In 1942, Cowan, Diehl, and Baker published an account in the *Journal of the American Medical Association* of a study that they had made of the incidence of colds in students in the University of Minnesota during the winter of 1939-1940.* The students had volunteered to participate in the study because they were particularly susceptible to colds. About four-hundred

---

*This is the study mentioned, rather inaccurately, by Dr. Fredrick J. Stare in the 1969 *Mademoiselle* article, and described by him as "a very careful study" (see the Introduction).

students participated in the study. About half of them received vitamin C, usually two 100-mg tablets per day, for a total of twenty-eight weeks, and the other half received a placebo. These students did not know that they were serving as controls.

The investigators concluded that this amount of ascorbic acid, about 200 mg per day, did not have an important effect on the number or severity of infections of the upper respiratory tract when administered to young adults who presumably were already on a reasonably adequate diet. They obtained, however, three results that seem to have significance. First, the average number of colds per person receiving ascorbic acid during the period of twenty-eight weeks was 1.9 ± 0.07, whereas the average number of colds in the control group was 2.2 ± 0.08. (Cowan, Diehl, and Baker should have reported their results to one more significant figure.) The investigators conclude that "the actual difference between the two groups during the year of the study amounts to 1/3 of a cold per person. Statistical analysis of the data reveals that a difference as large as this would arise only three or four times in a hundred through chance alone. One may therefore consider this as probably a significant difference, and vitamin C supplements to the diet may therefore be judged to give a slight advantage in reducing the number of colds experienced. However, one may well question the practical importance of such a difference."

This difference, one third, represents a decrease in the number of colds during the winter by 15 percent, 0.33/2.2, apparently resulting from ingestion of 200 mg of ascorbic acid per day. I think that such a difference does have practical importance. Also, the investigators might have asked whether taking twice as much ascorbic acid, 400 mg per day, would have decreased the number of colds by twice as much, 30 percent.

There is a second interesting aspect of the study made by Cowan, Diehl, and Baker. The ascorbic-acid group began with 233 students, of whom 25 dropped out during the twenty-eight weeks of the study. The control group began with 194 students, of whom 39 dropped out. Thus 20 percent of the control group dropped out of the study, and only 10 percent of those receiving ascorbic acid. The chance that this difference in the fraction of dropouts would occur in two samples of a uniform population is only 1 percent. Hence it seems likely that the population was not uniform in this respect; instead, a larger fraction of the students receiving ascorbic acid felt that they were benefited by the treatment than of those receiving the placebo.

A third aspect of the study is also statistically significant. The students who received the placebo lost an average of 1.6 days from school because of colds, and those who received ascorbic acid lost only an average of 1.1 days, 30 percent less. The probability that this difference would occur in a uniform population is only 0.1 percent.

A somewhat similar study, carried out in Scotland, was reported in 1942 by Glazebrook and Thomson. This study was carried out in an institution where there were about 1500 students, whose ages ranged from fifteen to twenty years. The food was poorly prepared, being kept hot for two hours or more before serving, and the total intake of ascorbic acid was determined to be only about 5 mg to 15 mg per student per day. Some of the students (335) were given additional ascorbic acid, 200 mg per day, for a period of six months, with the others (1100) kept as controls.

The incidence of colds and tonsilitis was 30.1 percent in the ascorbic-acid group during this period, and that in the controls was 34.5 percent. Thus there were 13 percent fewer colds among the students given ascorbic acid than among the controls, approximately the same decrease as was found in the Minnesota study, but with smaller statistical reliability (12 percent probability in a uniform population).

Students with moderately severe colds or tonsilitis were admitted to the Sick Quarters of the institution. Of the students receiving ascorbic acid 23.0 percent were admitted to Sick Quarters, as compared with 30.5 percent of the controls. Accordingly the number of serious cases of colds or tonsilitis, requiring admission to Sick Quarters, was 25 percent less for the students receiving ascorbic acid than for the controls. This difference has high statistical significance (only 1 percent probability in a uniform population).

The average number of days of hospitalization per student because of infection (common cold, tonsilitis, acute rheumatism, pneumonia) was 2.5 for the students receiving ascorbic acid and 5.0 for the controls. There were 17 cases of pneumonia and 16 cases of acute rheumatism among the 1100 controls, and no case of either disease among the 335 students receiving ascorbic acid. The probability of such a great difference in two samples of a uniform population is so small (less than 0.3 percent) as to indicate very strongly that ascorbic acid has value in providing protection against these serious infectious diseases, as well as against the common cold and tonsilitis.

Another study involving about the same amount of ascorbic acid per day was reported in 1956 by Franz, Sands, and Heyl. These investigators studied 89 volunteer medical students and student nurses for a period of three months, February to May 1956. A group of 44 subjects received ascorbic acid in the amount 195 mg per day, and 45 received no ascorbic acid. The number of colds was nearly the same, 14 for the ascorbic-acid group and 15 for the other group. The colds were less severe for the first group; only one cold lasted longer than five days for the ascorbic-acid group, as compared with eight for the control group.

The investigators concluded that "in this small series, those receiving ascorbic acid showed more rapid improvement in their colds than those not receiving it . . . statistically significant at the 0.05 level."

Another report on ascorbic acid and upper respiratory inflammation was published by Wilson and Low in 1970. These investigators carried out a double-blind trial with 103 subjects in a girls' school in Ireland. Of the subjects, 57 received 200 mg of ascorbic acid per day and 46 received placebo tablets, during several months of the winter. It was found that ascorbic acid reduced the incidence, duration, and severity of the symptoms of both toxic colds (sore throat, headache, fever, malaise) and catarrhal colds (cold in the head, cough, nasal obstruction, nasal discharge). Duration of the symptoms in catarrhal colds was reduced from 14 days to 8 days in the children receiving ascorbic acid. The concentration of ascorbic acid in the white blood cells of the girls who had received 200 mg per day for three months was 60 micrograms per hundred million cells, as compared with 43 micrograms per hundred million cells for the girls receiving the placebo tablets. This increase may be in part responsible for the increased resistance to infection.

A somewhat larger intake of ascorbic acid provides somewhat greater protection. A Swiss investigator, Dr. G. Ritzel, reported in 1961 the results of a double-blind study of the effect of five times as much as in the foregoing studies. He studied 279 skiers, half of whom received 1000 mg of ascorbic acid per day and the other half an identical inert placebo. He reported a reduction of 61 percent in the number of days of illness from upper respiratory infections and a reduction of 65 percent in the incidence of individual symptoms in the vitamin C group as compared with the placebo group. These results have high statistical significance (probability in two samples of a uniform population only 0.1 percent).*

The several studies made with administration of 200 mg of ascorbic acid per day over a considerable period of time indicate that this small amount of ascorbic acid has some value, decreasing the incidence of colds by about 15 percent. The report by Ritzel indicates that the ingestion of a larger amount of ascorbic acid, 1 g per day, has a greater protective power, decreasing the incidence by about 60 percent.

The evidence summarized above shows that even these small amounts, 200 mg to 1 g, of ascorbic acid, taken regularly, have some value in providing protection against the common cold.

In recent years a number of scientists and physicians have reported that the common cold can be almost completely controlled by use of still larger amounts of ascorbic acid, several grams per day. The leader in the ascorbic-acid field is Dr. Irwin Stone, a biochemist in Staten Island, New York. Dr. Stone published his first paper on ascorbic acid in 1935, and he has continued his investigations of the substance up to the present time. His principal thesis has been that the optimum intake of this important food by human beings is from 3 g to 5 g per day, rather than the far smaller amount, about 60 mg per day, recommended as the daily dietary allowance by the Food and Nutrition Board of the National Research Council.

---

*A serious error in reporting the results of this investigation was made by the author of the editorial article in *Nutrition Reviews* (1967), where it is stated that there was only 39 percent reduction in the number of days of illness and 35 percent reduction in the incidence of symptoms. This error may have contributed to the unfavorable opinion expressed in the article.

One way in which Dr. Stone reached this conclusion is by the study of the amounts of ascorbic acid present in the tissues of other animals. The gorilla requires ascorbic acid as a vitamin, as does man. In 1949 the British biochemist G. H. Bourne pointed out that the food ingested by the gorilla consists largely of fresh vegetation, in quantity such as to give the gorilla about 4.5 g of ascorbic acid per day, and that before the development of agriculture man existed largely on green plants, supplemented with some meat. He concluded that "it may be possible, therefore, that when we are arguing whether 7 or 30 mg of vitamin C a day is an adequate intake we may be very wide of the mark. Perhaps we should be arguing whether 1 g or 2 g a day is the correct amount." Stone (1966a) quoted this, and supplemented it by consideration of the rate of manufacture of ascorbic acid by the rat, which is the only animal for which this rate has been measured. The rat under normal conditions is reported to synthesize ascorbic acid at a rate between 26 mg per day per kilogram of body weight (Burns, Mosbach, and Schulenberg, 1954) and 58 mg per day per kilogram of body weight (Salomon and Stubbs, 1961). If the assumption is made that the same rate of production would be proper for a human being, a person weighing 70 kg (154 pounds) should ingest between 1.8 g and 4.1 g per day under ordinary circumstances. In one of his papers (1966b) Stone wrote that he himself has ingested 3 g to 5 g of ascorbic acid daily for the past ten years. He stated that during a period of ten years on this regimen he had not suffered a single common cold. In the statement about the high-level ascorbic-acid regimen that he sent me in 1966 Dr. Stone recommended 1.5 g (one-third of a level teaspoon of ascorbic acid powder) as a standard dose, to be dissolved in orange juice or tomato juice or in water, perhaps sweetened to taste. His recommended procedure for aborting a cold is that a dose of 1.5 g of ascorbic acid be taken at the first sign of development of the symptoms of a cold. Another dose is to be taken within an hour, and this is to be repeated at about one-hour intervals. Dr. Stone stated that usually by the third dose the cold is completely aborted, so that it does not develop. He warned that to be successful this procedure should be started at the very first indication of the cold.

The physician Edmé Régnier of Salem, Massachusetts, reported in 1968 that he had discovered the value of the administration of large doses of ascorbic acid in the prevention and treatment of the common cold. For many years, beginning at the age of seven, he had suffered from repeated bouts of inflammation of the middle ear. He had tried a number of ways of controlling the infections, and after twenty years he made a trial of the bioflavonoids (vitamin P complex, from citrus fruits) and ascorbic acid. He felt that this treatment had been of some benefit, but not very great. He decided to try increasing the amount. After several trials he found that the serious and disagreeable manifestations of the common cold and the accompanying inflammation of the middle ear could be averted by the use of large amounts of ascorbic acid, and that ascorbic acid alone was just as effective as the same amount of ascorbic acid plus bioflavonoids. He initiated a study of 22 subjects with use of ascorbic acid alone, ascorbic acid plus bioflavonoids, bioflavonoids alone, or a placebo. This study extended over a period of five years. At first the subjects were kept ignorant of the preparations that they received, but later on it became impossible to continue the blind study, because a patient whose cold was developing recognized that he was not receiving the vitamin C that might have prevented it.

The method of treatment recommended by Dr. Régnier is the administration of 600 mg of ascorbic acid at the first signs of a cold (scratchiness of the throat, nasal secretion, sneezing, a chill), followed by an additional 600 mg every three hours, or 200 mg of ascorbic acid every hour. At bedtime the amount ingested is increased to 750 mg. This intake, amounting to about 4 g of ascorbic acid per day, is to be continued for three or four days, reduced to 400 mg every three hours for several days, and then to 200 mg every three hours. Dr. Régnier reported that of 34 colds treated with ascorbic acid plus bioflavonoids, 31 were averted, and of 50 colds treated with ascorbic acid alone, as described above, 45 were averted. He had no success in treating colds with bioflavonoids alone, or with a placebo.

An important observation made by Dr. Régnier is that a cold that has been apparently aborted by the use of a large intake of ascorbic acid may return, even after a week or more, if the ingestion of ascorbic acid is suddenly discontinued.

A number of interesting comments about ascorbic acid and the common cold were made by Douglas Gildersleeve, M.D.,* in his article "Why Organized Medicine Sneezes at the Common Cold," published in the July-August 1967 issue of *Fact* magazine. In this article Dr. Gildersleeve stated that "having worked as a researcher in the field, it is my contention that effective treatment for the common cold, a cure, is available, that is being ignored because of the monetary losses that would be inflicted on pharmaceutical manufacturers, professional journals, and doctors themselves."

He wrote that he had found that he could suppress the symptoms of the common cold by making use of twenty or twenty-five times as much ascorbic acid as had been used by previous investigators, such as Tebrock, Arminio, and Johnston

---

*This name is probably a pseudonym, assumed by the author for professional reasons.

(Appendix III), who had used 200 mg per day. He reported that in studies carried out on more than 400 colds in 25 individuals, mostly his own patients, he had found the treatment with ascorbic acid in large amounts to be effective in 95 percent of the patients. The most frequent cold symptom, excessive nasal discharge, disappeared entirely on use of ascorbic acid, and other symptoms, sneezing, coughing, sore throat, hoarseness, and headache, were barely noticeable, if they were present at all. He reported that not one of the subjects ever experienced any secondary bacterial complications.

Dr. Gildersleeve reported in his *Fact* article that in 1964 he wrote a paper in which he described his observations. He submitted the paper to eleven different professional journals, every one of which rejected it. Dr. Gildersleeve also reported in his *Fact* article that one editor said to him that it would be harmful to the journal to publish a useful treatment for the common cold. He stated that medical journals depend for their existence on the support of their advertisers, and that over twenty-five percent of the advertisements in the journals relate to patented drugs for the alleviation of cold symptoms or for the treatment of complications of colds.

Another editor said that he had rejected the paper because it was not correct. When Dr. Gildersleeve questioned him about this statement, he said, "Twenty-five years ago I was a member of a team of researchers that investigated vitamin C. We determined then that the drug was of no use in treating the common cold." He was not impressed when Dr. Gildersleeve told him that the amount of ascorbic acid that had been used in the early work was only one-twentieth of the minimum amount necessary to achieve significant results.

I think that this anecdote explains in part the slowness with which the value of ascorbic acid has been recognized by the medical profession, except as a means of preventing scurvy. Since a very small intake, about 10 mg of ascorbic acid per day, is enough to prevent scurvy from developing in most human beings, 200 mg per day seems to be a large quantity, and accordingly most of the studies that have been carried out on the possible value of ascorbic acid in controlling the common cold have been restricted to quantities of this magnitude. The possibility that the optimum rate of intake of this important food, ascorbic acid, might be much larger than 200 mg per day has been recognized only during recent years.

In April 1970 I wrote to Dr. Albert Szent-Györgyi, who is the man who had first separated ascorbic acid from the plant and animal tissues in which it occurs, and who is now in the Laboratory of the Institute for Muscle Research, Woods Hole, Massachusetts. I asked his opinion about ascorbic acid, especially with relation to the optimum rate of intake. He has given me permission to quote part of his answering letter, as follows:

> As to ascorbic acid, right from the beginning I felt that the medical profession misled the public. If you don't take ascorbic acid with your food you get scurvy, so the medical profession said that if you don't get scurvy you are all right. I think that this is a very grave error. Scurvy is not the first sign of the deficiency but a premortal syndrome, and for full health you need much more, very much more. I am taking, myself, about 1 g a day. This does not mean that this is really the optimum dose because we do not know what full health really means and how much ascorbic acid you need for it. What I can tell you is that one can take any amount of ascorbic acid without the least danger.

It may be a long time before we know what the optimum rate of intake of this important food is. There is no doubt that it varies somewhat from person to person, as discussed in Chapter 8. I am sure that an increased intake of ascorbic acid, 10 to 100 times the daily allowance recommended by the Food and Nutrition Board, leads to improvement in general health and to increased resistance to infectious disease, including the common cold.

It is often stated that more vitamin C than the Food and Nutrition Board's recommended intake of about 60 mg per day is just wasted, because it is eliminated from the body in the urine. For example, Dr. Fredrick J. Stare in his book *Eating for Good Health* (1969) writes "But an extra amount of the vitamin cannot be stored in the body and is simply excreted." This argument is fallacious. In fact, a steady state is set up in the body such that the concentration of ascorbic acid in the blood is approximately proportional to the rate of intake. If you increase your intake tenfold, the concentration in the blood will become ten times as great.

In this chapter I have discussed some of the investigations that have been carried out on ascorbic acid in relation to the common cold; others are discussed in Appendix III. Some of these investigations have been well designed but, unfortunately, have involved the use of rather small quantities of ascorbic acid, and have shown only that these rather small quantities have limited value in preventing or ameliorating the common cold. So far as I am aware, no large-scale study, involving several hundred or thousand subjects, has been carried out to show to what extent the regular ingestion of ascorbic acid in large amounts is effective in preventing and ameliorating the common cold and associated infections. I hope that some such large-scale studies will be carried out; but in the meantime I am convinced by the evidence already available that ascorbic acid is to be preferred to the analgesics, antihistamines, and other dangerous drugs that are recommended for the treatment of the common cold by the purveyors of drugs.

Every day, even every hour, radio and television commercials extol various cold remedies. I hope that, as the results of further studies become available, extensive educational efforts about vitamin C and the common cold will be instituted on radio and television, including warnings against the use of dangerous drugs, like those about the hazards of smoking that are now sponsored by the United States Public Health Service, the American Cancer Society, the Heart Association, and other agencies.

Vitamin C and Evolution

A human being requires many different foods in order to be in good health. In addition to carbohydrates, proteins, essential fats, and minerals, he requires ascorbic acid and a number of other vitamins.

The protein in our diet is the principal source of the nitrogen required for the nitrogenous substances in our body, proteins and nucleic acids.

The proteins in the human body, and in other living organisms, are linear chains of residues of about twenty different amino acids—glycine, alanine, serine, lysine, phenylalanine, and fifteen others. It is not necessary that all of the amino acids be present in the diet. Some of them can be synthesized in the human body. But eight amino acids, called the essential amino acids, cannot be synthesized in the human body, and must be present in the food that is ingested. The eight essential amino acids are threonine, valine, methionine, lysine, histidine, phenylalanine, tryptophan, and leucine. The disease kwashiorkor (protein starvation) results from an inadequate intake of the essential amino acids.

We are accustomed to thinking of man as the highest of all species of living organisms. In one sense he is: he has achieved effective control over a large part of the earth, and has even begun to extend his realm as far as the moon. But in his biochemical capabilities he is inferior to many other organisms, including even unicellular organisms, such as bacteria, yeasts, and molds.

The red bread mold (*Neurospora*), for example, is able to carry out in its cells a great many chemical reactions that human beings are unable to carry out. The red bread mold can live on a very simple medium, consisting of water, inorganic salts, an inorganic source of nitrogen, such as ammonium nitrate, a suitable source of carbon, such as sucrose, and a single "vitamin," biotin. All other substances required by the red bread mold are synthesized by it, with use of its internal mechanisms. The red bread mold does not need to have any amino acids in its diet, because it is able to synthesize all of them, and also to synthesize all of the vitamins except biotin.

The red bread mold owes its survival, over hundreds of millions of years, to its great biochemical capabilities. If, like man, it were unable to synthesize the various amino acids and vitamins it would not have survived, because it could not have solved the problem of getting an adequate diet.

From time to time a gene in the red bread mold undergoes a mutation, such as to cause the cell to lose the ability to manufacture one of the amino acids or vitamin-like substances essential to its life. This mutated spore gives rise to a deficient strain of red bread mold, which could stay in good health only with an addition to the diet that suffices for the original type of the mold. The scientists G. W. Beadle and E. L. Tatum carried on extensive studies of mutated strains of the red bread mold, when they were working in Stanford University, beginning about 1938. They were able to keep the mutant strains alive in the laboratory by providing each strain with the additional food that it needed for good health, as shown by a normal rate of growth.

It was mentioned in Chapter 3 that the substance thiamine (vitamin B_1) is needed by human beings to keep them from dying of the disease beriberi, and that chickens fed on a diet that contains none of this food also die of a neurological disease resembling beriberi. It has been found, in fact, that thiamine is needed as an essential food for all other animal species that have been studied, including the domestic pigeon, the laboratory rat, the guinea pig, the pig, the cow, the domestic cat, and the monkey.

We may surmise that the need of all of these animal species for thiamine as an essential food, which they must ingest in order not to develop a disease resembling beriberi in human beings, resulted from an event that took place over 500 million years ago. Let us consider the epoch, early in the history of life on earth, when the early animal species from which present-day birds and mammals have evolved populated a part of the earth. We assume that the animals of this species nourished themselves by eating plants, possibly together with other food. Many plants contain thiamine. Accordingly the animals would have in their bodies thiamine that they had ingested with the foodstuffs that they had eaten, as well as the thiamine that they themselves synthesized by use of their own synthetic mechanism. Now let us assume that a mutant animal appeared in the population, an animal that, as the result of impact of a cosmic ray on a gene or of the action of some other mutagenic agent, had lost the biochemical machinery that still permitted the other members of the species to manufacture thiamine from other substances. The amount of thiamine provided by the ingestion of food would suffice to keep the mutant well nourished, essentially as well nourished as the unmutated animals; and the mutant would have an advantage over the unmutated animals, in that it would be liberated of the burden of the machinery for manufacturing its own thiamine. As a result the mutant would be able to have more offspring than the other animals in the population. By reproduction the mutated animal would pass its advantageously mutated gene along to some of its offspring, and they too would have more than the average number of offspring. Thus in the course of time this advantage, the advantage of not having to do the work of manufacturing thiamine or to carry within itself the machinery for this manufacture, could permit the mutant type to replace the original type.

Many different kinds of molecules must be present in the body of an animal in order that the animal be in good health. Some of these molecules can be synthesized by the animal; others must be ingested as foods. If the substance is available as a food, it is advantageous to the animal species to rid itself of the burden of the machinery for synthesizing it.

It is believed that, over the millenia, the ancestors of human beings were enabled, over and over again, by the availability of certain substances as foods, including the essential amino acids and the vitamins, to simplify their own biochemical lives by shuffling off the machinery that had been needed by their ancestors for synthesizing these substances. It is evolutionary processes of this sort that gradually, over periods of millions of years, led to the appearance of new species, including man.

Some very interesting experiments have been carried out on competition between strains of organisms that require a certain substance as food and those that do not require the substance, because of the ability to synthesize it themselves. These experiments were carried out in the University of California, Los Angeles, by Zamenhof and Eichhorn, who published their findings in 1967. They studied a bacterium, *Bacillus subtilis*, by comparing a strain that had the power of manufacturing the amino acid tryptophan and a mutant strain that had lost the ability to manufacture this amino acid. If the same numbers of cells of the two strains were put in a medium that did not contain any tryptophan, the strain that could manufacture tryptophan survived, whereas the other strain died out. If, however, some cells of the two strains were put together in a medium containing a good supply of tryptophan the scales were turned: the mutant strain, which had lost the ability to manufacture the amino acid, survived, and the original strain, with the ability to manufacture the amino acid, died out. The two strains of bacteria differed only in a single mutation, the loss of the ability to manufacture the amino acid tryptophan. We are hence led to conclude that the burden of using the machinery for tryptophan synthesis was disadvantageous to the strain possessing this ability, and hampered it, in its competition with the mutant strain, to such an extent as to cause it to fail in this competition. The number of generations (cell divisions) required for take-over in this series of experiments (starting with an equal number of cells, to a million times as many cells of the victorious strain) was about fifty, which would correspond to only about 1500 years for man (30 years per generation).

We may say that Zamenhof and Eichhorn carried out a small-scale experiment about the process of the evolution of species. This experiment, and several others that they also carried out, showed that it can be advantageous to be free of the internal machinery for synthesizing a vital substance, if the vital substance can be obtained instead as a food from the immediate environment.

Most of the vitamins required by man for good health are also required by animals of other species. Vitamin A is an essential nutrient for all vertebrates for vision, maintenance of skin tissue, and normal development of bones. Riboflavin (vitamin B_2), pantothenic acid, pyridoxine (vitamin B_6), nicotinic acid (niacin), and cyanocobalamin (vitamin B_{12}) are required for good health by the cow, pig, rat, chicken, and other animals. It is likely that the loss of the ability to synthesize these essential substances, like the loss of the ability to synthesize thiamine, occurred rather early in the history of life on earth, when the primitive animals began living largely on plants, which contain a supply of these nutrients.

Dr. Irwin Stone pointed out in 1965 that, whereas most species of animals can synthesize ascorbic acid, man and other primates that have been tested, including the rhesus monkey, the Formosan long tail monkey, and the ringtail or brown capuchin monkey, are unable to synthesize the substance, and require it as a vitamin. He concluded that the loss of the ability to synthesize ascorbic acid probably occurred in the common ancestor of the primates. A rough estimate of the time at which this mutational change occurred is twenty-five million years ago (Zuckerkandl and Pauling, 1962).

The guinea pig and an Indian fruit-eating bat are the only other mammals known to require ascorbic acid as a vitamin. The red-vented bulbul and some other Indian birds (of the order Passeriformes) also require ascorbic acid. The overwhelming majority of mammals, birds, amphibians, and reptiles have the ability to synthesize the substance in their tissues, usually in the liver or the kidney. The loss of the ability by the guinea pig, the fruit-eating bat, and the red-vented bulbul and some other species of passeriform birds probably resulted from independent mutations in populations of these species of animals living in an environment that provided an ample supply of ascorbic acid in the available foodstuffs.

We may ask why ascorbic acid is not required as a vitamin in the food of the cow, pig, horse, rat, chicken, and many other species of animals that do require the other vitamins required by man. Ascorbic acid is present in green plants, along with these other vitamins. When green plants became the steady diet of the common ancestor of man and other mammals, hundreds of millions of years ago, why did not this ancestor undergo the mutation of eliminating the mechanism for synthesizing ascorbic acid, as well as the mechanisms for synthesizing thiamine, pantothenic acid, pyridoxine, and other vitamins?

I think that the answer to this question is that for optimum health more ascorbic acid was needed than could be provided under ordinary conditions by the usually available green plants.

Let us consider the common precursor of the primates, at a time about twenty-five million years ago. This animal and his ancestors had for hundreds of millions of years continued to synthesize ascorbic acid from other substances that they had ingested. Let us assume that a population of this species of animals was living, at that time, in an area that provided an ample supply of food with an unusually large content of ascorbic acid, permitting the animals to obtain from their diet approximately the amount of ascorbic acid needed for optimum health. A cosmic ray or some other mutagenic agent then caused a mutation to occur, such that the enzyme in the liver that catalyzes the conversion of L-gulonolactone to ascorbic acid was no longer present in the liver. Some of the progeny of this mutant animal would have inherited the loss of the ability to synthesize ascorbic acid. These mutant animals would, in the environment that provided an ample supply of ascorbic acid, have an advantage over the ascorbic-acid-producing animals, in that they had been relieved of the burden of constructing and operating the machinery for producing ascorbic acid. Under these conditions the mutant would gradually replace the earlier strain.

A mutation that involves the loss of the ability to synthesize an enzyme occurs often. Such a mutation requires only that the gene be damaged in some way or be deleted. (The reverse mutation, leading to the ability to produce the enzyme, is difficult, and would occur only extremely rarely.) Once the ability to synthesize ascorbic acid has been lost by a species of animals, that species depends for its existence on the availability of ascorbic acid as a food.

The fact that most species of animals have not lost the ability to manufacture their own ascorbic acid shows that the supply of ascorbic acid available generally in foodstuffs is not sufficient to provide the optimum amount of this substance. Only in an unusual environment, in which the available food provided unusually large amounts of ascorbic acid, have circumstances permitted a species of animal to abandon its own powers of synthesis of this important substance. These unusual circumstances occurred for the precursor of man and other primates, for the guinea pig, for the Indian fruit-eating bat, and for the precursor of the red-vented bulbul and some other species of passeriform birds, but have not occurred, through the hundreds of millions of years of evolution, for the precursors of the cow, the horse, the pig, the rat, and hundreds of other animals. Thus the consideration of evolutionary processes, as presented in the foregoing analysis, indicates that the ordinarily available foodstuffs might well provide essentially the optimum amounts of thiamine, riboflavin, niacin, vitamin A, and other vitamins that are required as essential nutrients by all mammalian species, but be deficient in ascorbic acid. For this food, essential for man but synthesized by many other species of animals, the optimum rate of intake is indicated to be larger than the rate associated with the ingestion of the ordinarily available diet.

I have checked the amounts of various vitamins present in 110 raw, natural plant foods, as given in the tables in the metabolism handbook published by the Federation of American Societies for Experimental Biology (Altman and Dittmer, 1968). When the amounts of vitamins corresponding to one day's food for an adult (the amount that provides 2500 kilocalories of energy) are calculated, it is found that for most vitamins this amount is about three times the daily allowance recommended by the Food and Nutrition Board. For ascorbic acid, however, the average amount in the daily ration of the 110 plant foodstuffs is 2.3 g, about forty-two times the amount recommended as the daily allowance for a person with a caloric requirement of 2500 kilocalories per day (see Table 1, on the following page).

If the need for ascorbic acid were really as small as the daily allowance recommended by the Food and Nutrition Board the mutation would surely have occurred 500 million years

TABLE 1

Vitamin Content of 110 Raw Natural Plant Foods
Referred to Amount Giving 2500 Kilocalories of Food Energy

Foods	Thiamine	Riboflavin	Niacin	Ascorbic acid
Nuts and grains (11)	3.2 mg	1.5 mg	27 mg	0 mg
Fruit, low C (21)	1.9	2.0	19	600
Beans and peas (15)	7.5	4.7	34	1000
Berries, low C (8)	1.7	2.0	15	1200
Vegetables, low C (25)	5.0	5.9	39	1200
Intermediate-C foods (16)	7.8	9.8	77	3400
High-C foods (6)	8.1	19.6	58	6000
Very high-C foods (8)	6.1	9.0	68	12000
Averages for 110 foods	5.0	5.4	41	2300
Recommended daily allowance for adult	1.0 to 1.6 mg	1.3 to 1.7 mg	13 to 20 mg	50 to 60 mg
Ratio of plant food average to average recommended allowance	3.8	3.6	2.5	42

Nuts and grains: almonds, filberts, macadamia nuts, peanuts, barley, brown rice, whole grain rice, sesame seeds, sunflower seeds, wheat, wild rice.

Fruit (low in vitamin C, less than 2500 mg): apples, apricots, avocadoes, bananas, cherries (sour red, sweet), coconut, dates, figs, grapefruit, grapes, kumquats, mangoes, nectarines, peaches, pears, pineapple, plums, crabapples, honeydew melon, watermelon.

Beans and peas: broad beans (immature seeds, mature seeds), cowpeas (immature seeds, mature seeds), lima beans (immature seeds, mature seeds), mung beans (seeds, sprouts), peas (edible pod, green mature seeds), snapbeans (green, yellow), soybeans (immature seeds, mature seeds, sprouts).

Berries (low C, less than 2500 mg): blackberries, blueberries, cranberries, loganberries, raspberries, currants (red), gooseberries, tangerines.

Vegetables (low C, less than 2500 mg): bamboo shoots, beets, carrots, celeriac root, celery, corn, cucumber, dandelion greens, egg-plant, garlic cloves, horseradish, lettuce, okra, onions (young, mature), parsnips, potatoes, pumpkins, rhubarb, rutabagas, squash (summer, winter), sweet potatoes, green tomatoes, yams.

Intermediate-C foods (2500 to 4900 mg): artichokes, asparagus, beet greens, cantaloupe, chicory greens, chinese cabbage, fennel, lemons, limes, oranges, radishes, spinach, zucchini, strawberries, swiss chard, ripe tomatoes.

High-C foods (5000 to 7900 mg): brussels sprouts, cabbage, cauliflower, chives, collards, mustard greens.

Very high-C foods (8000 to 16500 mg): broccoli spears, black currants, kale, parsley, hot chili peppers (green, red), sweet peppers (green, red).

ago, and dogs, cows, pigs, horses, and other animals would be obtaining ascorbic acid from their food, instead of manufacturing it in their own liver cells.

Therefore, I conclude that 2.3 g per day is less than the optimum rate of intake of ascorbic acid for an adult human being.

The average ascorbic-acid content of the fourteen plant foodstuffs richest in this vitamin is 9.4 g per 2500 kilocalories. Peppers (hot or sweet, green or red) and black currants are richest of all, with 15 g per 2500 kilocalories. These amounts indicate an upper limit for the optimum daily intake for man.

I conclude that the optimum daily intake of ascorbic acid for most adult human beings lies in the range 2.3 g to 9 g. The amount of individual biochemical variability (Chapter 8) is such that for a large population the range may be as great as from 250 mg to 10 g or more per day.

The foregoing argument represents an extension and refinement of Bourne's gorilla argument, and it leads to a similar conclusion. The conclusion about the optimum intake is also nearly the same as that from Stone's rat argument (1.8 g to 4.1 g per day).

It is, of course, almost certain that some evolutionarily effective mutations have occurred in man and his immediate predecessors rather recently (within the last few million years) such as to permit life to continue on an intake of ascorbic acid less than that provided by high-ascorbic-acid raw plant foods. These mutations might involve an increased ability of the kidney tubules to pump ascorbic acid back into the blood from the glomerular filtrate (dilute urine, being concentrated on passage along the tubules) and an increased ability of certain cells to extract ascorbic acid from the blood plasma. It is likely that the adrenal glands act as a storehouse of ascorbic acid, extracting it from the blood when green plant foods are available, in the summer, and releasing it slowly when the supply is depleted. On general principles we can conclude, however, that these mechanisms require energy and are a burden to the organism. The optimum rate of intake of ascorbic acid might still be within the range given above, 2.3 g per day or more, or might be somewhat less; and, of course, there is always the factor of biochemical individuality, discussed in Chapter 8.

CHAPTER 7

Orthomolecular Medicine

Orthomolecular medicine is the preservation of good health and the treatment of disease by varying the concentrations in the human body of substances that are normally present in the body and are required for health (Pauling, 1968).

Death by starvation, kwashiorkor, beriberi, scurvy, or any other deficiency disease can be averted by the provision of an adequate daily intake of carbohydrates, essential fats, proteins (including the essential amino acids), essential minerals, thiamine, ascorbic acid, and other vitamins. To achieve the best of health, the rate of intake of essential foods should be such as to establish and maintain the optimum concentrations of essential molecules, such as those of ascorbic acid. There is no doubt that a high concentration of ascorbic acid is needed to provide the maximum protection against infection, and to permit the rapid healing of wounds. I believe that in general the treatment of disease by the use of substances, such as ascorbic acid, that are normally present in the human body and are required for life is to be preferred to the treatment by the use of powerful synthetic substances or plant products, which may, and usually do, have undesirable side effects.

An example of orthomolecular medicine is the treatment of diabetes mellitus by the injection of insulin. Diabetes mellitus is a hereditary disease, usually caused by a recessive gene. The hereditary defect results in a deficient production by the pancreas of the hormone insulin. The primary effect of insulin is to cause an increase in the rate of extraction of glucose from the blood. In the absence of insulin the concentration of glucose in the blood of the patient becomes much greater than normal, resulting in the manifestations of the disease.

Insulin extracted from cattle pancreas or pig pancreas differs only slightly in its molecular structure from human insulin, and it has essentially the same physiological activity. The injection of cattle insulin or pig insulin is essentially the provision of the normal concentration of insulin in the body of the patient; it permits the metabolism of glucose to take place at the normal rate, and thus serves to counteract the abnormality resulting from the genetic defect. Insulin therapy is accordingly an example of orthomolecular therapy. Its major disadvantage is that the insulin cannot be introduced into the blood stream except by injection.

Another way in which the disease can be kept under control, if it is not serious, is by adjusting the diet, regulating the intake of sugar, in such a way as to keep the glucose concentration in the blood within the normal limits. This procedure also represents an example of orthomolecular medicine.

A third procedure, the use of so-called oral insulin, a drug taken by mouth, does not constitute an example of orthomolecular medicine, because oral insulin is a synthetic drug, foreign to the human body, and it may have undesirable side effects.

Another disease that is treated by orthomolecular methods is phenylketonuria. Phenylketonuria results from a genetic defect that leads to a decreased amount or effectiveness of an enzyme in the liver which in normal persons catalyzes the oxidation of one amino acid, phenylalanine, to another, tyrosine. Ordinary proteins contain several percent of phenylalanine, providing a much larger amount of this amino acid than a person needs. The concentration of phenylalanine in the blood and other body fluids of the patient becomes abnormally high, if he is on a normal diet, causing the manifestations of the disease: mental deficiency, severe eczema, and others. The disease can be controlled by use, beginning in infancy, of a diet that contains a smaller amount of phenylalanine than is present in ordinary foods. In this way the concentration of phenylalanine in the blood and other body fluids is kept to approximately the normal level, and the manifestations of the disease do not appear.

A somewhat similar disease, which can also be controlled by orthomolecular methods, is galactosemia. Galactosemia involves the failure to manufacture an enzyme that carries out the metabolism of galactose, which is a part of milk sugar (lactose). The disease manifests itself in mental retardation, cataracts, cirrhosis of the liver and spleen, and nutritional failure. These manifestations are averted by placing the infant on a diet free of milk sugar, with the result that the concentration of galactose in the blood does not exceed the normal limit.

A conceivable sort of orthomolecular therapy for a hereditary disease involving a defective gene would be to introduce the gene (molecules of DNA, deoxyribonucleic acid), separated from the tissues of another person, into the cells of the person suffering from the disease. For example, some molecules of the gene that directs the synthesis of the enzyme that catalyzes the oxidation of phenylalanine to tyrosine could be separated from liver cells of a normal human being and introduced into the liver cells of a person with phenylketonuria. This sort of change in genetic character of an organism has been carried out for microorganisms, but not yet for human beings, and it is not likely that it will become an important way of controlling genetic defects until many decades have passed.

Another possible method of orthomolecular therapy for phenylketonuria, resembling the use of insulin in controlling diabetes, would be the injection of the active enzyme. There are two reasons why this treatment has not been developed. First, although it is known that the enzyme is present in the liver of animals, including man, it has not yet been isolated in purified form. Second, the natural mechanism of immunity, which involves the action of antibodies against proteins foreign to the species, would operate to destroy the enzyme prepared from the liver of animals of another species. This mechanism in general prevents the use of enzymes or other proteins from animals other than man in the treatment of diseases of human beings. Insulin is an exceptional protein, in that the molecules are unusually small. The insulin molecule contains polypeptide chains of two kinds, one containing 21 amino-acid residues and the other containing 30, whereas the polypeptide chains of most proteins contain between 100 and 200 residues. The structural difference between human insulin and animal insulin is very small; for example, pig insulin differs from human insulin in only one residue of the total of 51. This difference is so small as not to invoke the production of antibodies.

There is still another possible type of orthomolecular therapy. The molecules of many enzymes consist of two parts: the pure protein part, called the apoenzyme, and a non-protein part, called the coenzyme. The active enzyme, called the holoenzyme, is the apoenzyme with the coenzyme attached to it. Often the coenzyme is a vitamin molecule or a closely related molecule. It is known, for example, that a number of different enzymes in the human body, catalyzing different chemical reactions, have thiamine pyrophosphate, a derivative of thiamine (vitamin B_1), as coenzyme.

In some cases of genetic disease the enzyme is not absent, but is present with diminished activity. One way in which the defective gene can operate is to produce an apoenzyme with abnormal structure, such that it does not combine readily with the coenzyme to form the active enzyme. Under ordinary physiological conditions, with the normal concentration of coenzyme, perhaps only one percent of the abnormal apoenzyme has combined with the coenzyme. According to the principles of chemical equilibrium, a larger fraction of the abnormal apoenzyme could be made to combine with the coenzyme by increasing the concentration of the coenzyme in the body fluids. If the concentration were to be increased one hundred times, most of the apoenzyme molecules might combine with the coenzyme, to give essentially the normal amount of active enzyme.

There is accordingly the possibility that the disease could be kept under control by the ingestion by the patient of a very large amount of the vitamin that serves as a coenzyme. This sort of orthomolecular therapy, involving only a substance normally present in the human body (the vitamin), is, in my opinion, the preferable therapy.

An example of a disease that might be controlled in this way is the disease methylmalonicaciduria. The patients with this disease are deficient in the active enzyme that catalyzes the conversion of a simple substance, methylmalonic acid, to succinic acid. It is known that cyanocobalamin (vitamin B_{12})

serves as the coenzyme for this reaction. It is found that the provision of very large amounts of vitamin B_{12}, giving concentrations about a thousand times the normal concentration, causes the reaction to proceed at the normal rate for many of the patients.

The use of very large amounts of vitamins in the control of disease has been called megavitamin therapy. Megavitamin therapy is one aspect of orthomolecular medicine. It is my opinion that in the course of time it will be found possible to control hundreds of diseases by megavitamin therapy. For example, Dr. A. Hoffer and Dr. H. Osmond have reported that many patients with schizophrenia are benefited by megavitamin therapy. Their treatment, as was mentioned in the Introduction, includes the administration of nicotinic acid (niacin) or nicotinamide (niacinamide) in amounts of 3 g to 18 g per day, together with 3 g per day of ascorbic acid.

It is known that ascorbic acid is required for the synthesis of connective tissue. This fact provides an explanation for the reported value of large quantities of ascorbic acid in the treatment of rheumatoid arthritis and other connective-tissue diseases. Dr. Irwin Stone, in his discussion of the optimal rates of intake of ascorbic acid (1966), has written that "full 'correction' of the genetic defect, by keeping collagen synthesis and repair at optimal levels throughout lifetime, may produce an organism highly resistant to the rheumatoid disease process. This new concept also provides a basis for a rationale for the therapeutic use of ascorbic acid in these diseases at possibly 25 to 50 g per day or even higher." He also states that these doses can be administered without danger to the participants; "ascorbic acid is probably the least toxic of any known substance of comparable physiologic activity."

A large rate of intake of ascorbic acid is required for optimal protection against infectious disease. The use of ascorbic acid to provide protection against the common cold, influenza, rheumatic fever, pneumonia, and other infectious diseases may well be the most important of all methods of orthomolecular medicine.

CHAPTER 8

Human Biochemical Individuality

In considering the problem of protection against the common cold and other diseases we must recognize that human beings differ from one another. Professor Roger J. Williams, who for many years has been interested in the question of these differences (see his books *Biochemical Individuality*, 1956, and *You Are Extraordinary*, 1967), has pointed out that it is unlikely that any human being is exactly the "average" man.

Let us consider some character, such as the weight of the liver relative to the total weight of the human being, or the concentration of a certain enzyme in the red cells of the blood. It is found that, when a sample of 100 human beings is studied, this character varies over a several-fold range. The variation often is approximately that given by the standard bell-shaped probability function. It is customary to say that the "normal" range of values of the character is that range within which 95 percent of the values lie, and that the remaining 5 percent of the values, representing the extremes, are abnormal. If we assume that 500 characters are independently inherited, then we can calculate that there is only a small chance, 10 percent, that one person in the whole population of the world would be normal with respect to each of these 500 characters. But it is estimated that a human being has a complement of 100,000 genes, each of which serves some function, such as controlling the synthesis of an enzyme. The number of characters that can be variable, because of a difference in the nature of a particular gene, is presumably somewhere near 100,000, rather than only 500; and accordingly we reach the conclusion that no single human being on earth is normal (within the range that includes 95 percent of human beings) with respect to all characters. This calculation is, of course, oversimplified; but, as mentioned by Williams, it helps emphasize the point that human beings differ from one another, and that each human being must be treated as an individual.

The species Man is more heterogeneous, with respect to genetic character, than most other animal species. Nevertheless, heterogeneity has been found also for laboratory animals such as guinea pigs. It was recognized long ago that guinea pigs fed the same scurvy-producing diet, containing less than 5 mg of ascorbic acid per day per kilogram of body weight, differed in the severity of the scurvy that they developed and in the rapidity with which they developed it. A striking experiment was carried out in 1967 by Williams and Deason. These investigators obtained some male weanling guinea pigs from an animal dealer and, after a week of observation during which the guinea pigs were on a good diet, including fresh vegetables, they were placed on a diet free of ascorbic acid or with known amounts added. They were divided into eight groups, each of 10 to 15 guinea pigs, with one of the groups receiving no ascorbic acid and the other groups receiving varying amounts of ascorbic acid by mouth, given by pipet. About 80 percent of the animals receiving no ascorbic acid or only 0.5 mg per kilogram per day developed symptoms of scurvy, about 25 percent of those receiving between 1 mg and 4 mg per kilogram per day, and none of those receiving 8 mg per day or more. These results agree with the customary statement that about 5 mg per kilogram per day of ascorbic acid is required to prevent scurvy in guinea pigs.

It was observed, however, that two animals receiving only 1 mg per kilogram per day remained healthy and gained weight over the entire period of the experiment (eight weeks). One of them showed a total gain in weight larger than that for any animal receiving 2, 4, 8, or 16 times as much ascorbic acid.

On the other hand, seven of the guinea pigs receiving 8, 16, or 32 mg per kilogram per day were unhealthy, and showed very small growth during the first ten days on the diet. They were then provided with a larger amount of the vitamin, 5 of them with 64 mg per kilogram per day and 2 of them with 128 mg per kilogram per day. These animals showed a remarkable response: whereas they had grown only 12 grams, on the average, in a period of ten days on the smaller amounts of ascorbic acid, their growth during the ten-day period after beginning to receive the larger amounts was, on the average, 72 grams. The indicated conclusion is that these animals, 7 of the 30 that were placed on between 8 mg and 32 mg per kilogram per day, had a larger requirement of vitamin C for good health than the others. Williams and Deason reached the conclusion that there is at least a twenty-fold range in the vitamin-C needs of individual guinea pigs in a population of 100. They pointed out that the population of human beings is presumably not more uniform than that of the guinea pigs used in their experiments, and that accordingly the individual variation in human vitamin C needs is probably just as great.

I have accepted their conclusion, and similar conclusions reached by other investigators,* in suggesting that the optimum rate of intake of ascorbic acid by human beings may extend over a wide range, perhaps the forty-fold range from 250 mg per day to 10 g per day.

---

*There is some direct evidence about great variability in the intake of ascorbic acid required to prevent scurvy in human beings. Cochrane (1965) reported his observation of two infants with scurvy, in the Children's Hospital in Halifax, Nova Scotia. The physician questioned the parents and the pharmacy that had provided a vitamin preparation, and analyzed the preparation for ascorbic acid, finding it to have full potency. He concluded that the infants had each been receiving about 60 mg of ascorbic acid per day, and suggested that the ingestion of excessive amounts by the mother during pregnancy might "condition" the infant to requirements greater than the present expected or recommended intake. At the other extreme, DeJong, Robertson, and Schafer (1968) of Stanford University School of Medicine and Stanford Childrens Convalescent Hospital have reported that an infant with Hurler's syndrome was placed on a diet deficient in ascorbic acid at the age of ten weeks and has remained on this diet for a year without demonstrating any clinical or chemical evidence of scurvy, and with normal healing of a wound incurred during surgery for inguinal hernia. The intake of ascorbic acid was reported to have varied from 1.7 mg to 3.4 mg per day. (The patient was placed on this diet because of evidence that this serious congenital disease can be controlled to some extent by restricting the intake of ascorbic acid.) These cases correspond to a more than twenty-fold variation in the need for ascorbic acid to prevent scurvy.

CHAPTER 9

Vitamin C and Drugs Compared

Ascorbic acid, vitamin C, is a food—an essential food, required by human beings for life and good health. It is safe, even when taken in very large amounts, far larger than the amounts that are needed to combat the common cold. Some people may find it desirable to take it together with some other food, in order that it not have a laxative action; this suggestion is essentially the only warning that need be made. There is no reason to fear that children will harm themselves with ascorbic acid. Its sour taste is likely to keep a child from eating very much, and he would not become seriously ill even if he were to eat several spoonfuls. Ascorbic acid is described in reference books as essentially nontoxic. Animals receiving daily amounts that correspond to 350 g (over three-quarters of a pound) per day for a man developed no symptoms of toxicity. With respect to safety, ascorbic acid is ideal.

The drugs that are used in tremendous amounts for treating the common cold, and that are advertised to an irritatingly great extent on television and radio and in newspapers and magazines, are much different; they are harmful and dangerous, and are themselves responsible for much illness and many deaths.

Aspirin is the prime example. This drug, which is the chemical substance acetylsalicylic acid, is present in most cold medicines. The fatal dose for an adult is 20 g to 30 g. The ordinary aspirin tablet contains 324 mg (5 grains); hence 60 to 90 tablets can kill an adult, and a smaller amount can kill a child. Aspirin is the most common single poison used by suicides (it is second only to the group of substances used in sleeping pills). About 15 percent of accidental poisoning deaths of young children are caused by aspirin. Many lives would be saved if the medicine chest contained ascorbic acid in place of aspirin and the other cold medicines.

Some people show a severe sensitivity to aspirin, such that a decrease in circulation of the blood and difficulty in breathing follow the ingestion of 0.3 g to 1 g (one to three tablets).

The symptoms of mild aspirin poisoning are burning pain in the mouth, throat, and abdomen, difficulty in breathing, lethargy, vomiting, ringing in the ears, and dizziness. More severe poisoning leads to delirium, fever, sweating, incoordination, coma, convulsions, cyanosis (blueness of the skin), failure of kidney function, respiratory failure, and death.

Aspirin, like other salicylates, has the property that in concentrated solution it can attack and dissolve tissues. An aspirin tablet in the stomach may attack the stomach wall and cause the development of a bleeding ulcer.

There are several other substances closely related to aspirin that have analgesic properties (the ability to decrease the sensitivity to pain) and antipyretic properties (the ability to lower increased body temperature) and are present in some of the popular cold medicines. One of these is salicylamide (the amide of salicylic acid). It has about the same toxicity as aspirin: 20 g to 30 g is the lethal dose for an adult.

The closely related analgesic substances acetanilide (N-phenylacetamide), phenacetin (acetophenetidin), and acetaminophen (p-hydroxyacetanilide) are used alone or in combination with other drugs in a number of cold medicines, in amounts of 150 mg to 200 mg per tablet. These substances damage the liver and kidneys. A single dose of 0.5 g to 5 g may cause fall of blood pressure, failure of kidney function, and death by respiratory failure.

Many of the cold medicines available without prescription contain not only aspirin or some other analgesic but also an antihistamine and an antitussive (to control severe coughing). For example, one preparation, recommended on the box for "Fast temporary relief of cold symptoms and accompanying coughs, sinus congestion, headache, the symptoms of hay fever," contains in each tablet 12 mg of the antihistamine methapyrilene hydrochloride and 5 mg of the antitussive dextromethorphan hydrobromide, as well as some phenacetin, salicylamide, and other substances. In the *Handbook of Poisoning* (Dreisbach, 1969) it is reported that the death of a small child was caused by the estimated amount 100 mg of methapyrilene (114 mg of the hydrochloride). At least twenty deaths of children have resulted from accidental poisoning by antihistamines.

The estimated fatal dose for these reported poisonings lies in the range 10 mg to 50 mg per kilogram body weight for phenindamine, methapyrilene, diphenhydramine, and pyrilamine, and is probably about the same for many other antihistamines. These substances are more toxic than aspirin; one or two grams might cause the death of an adult.

These medicines often cause side effects, such as drowsiness and dizziness, even when taken in the recommended amounts. On the package there is usually a warning about the possibility of poisoning, for example,

> Keep this and all medicines out of children's
> reach. In case of accidental overdose, contact
> a physician immediately.

Moreover, there is often a more extensive warning, such as the following:

> CAUTION: Children under 12 should use only as directed by a physician. If symptoms persist or are unusually severe, see a physician. Do not exceed recommended dosage. Not for frequent or prolonged use. If excessive dryness of the mouth occurs, decrease dosage. Discontinue use if rapid pulse, dizziness, skin rash, or blurring of vision occurs. Do not drive or operate machinery as this preparation may cause drowsiness in some persons. Individuals with high blood pressure, heart disease, diabetes, thyroid disease, glaucoma or excessive pressure within the eye, and elderly persons (where undiagnosed glaucoma or excessive pressure within the eye may be present) should use only as directed by physician. Persons with undiagnosed glaucoma may experience eye pain; if this occurs discontinue use and see physician immediately.

The substance dextromethorphan hydrobromide, mentioned above as an antitussive, controls severe coughing by exerting a depressant effect on the brain. Also, the related substance codeine (as codeine phosphate) in amounts 15 mg to 30 mg every three or four hours is often prescribed by physicians for severe coughing. In most states of the United States codeine is not present in the medicines sold without prescription, but many of these medicines contain some other antitussive, such as dextromethorphan. The minimum fatal dose of these substances ranges from 100 mg to 1 g for an adult; much less for infants and more for narcotic addicts.

Some non-prescription cold medicines also contain belladonna alkaloids (atropine sulfate, hyoscyamine sulfate, scopolamine hydrobromide) in amounts as great as 0.2 mg per capsule. These drugs serve to dilate the bronchi and prevent spasms. They are intensely poisonous; the fatal dose in children may be as low as 10 mg. Side effects that may occur from ordinary doses are abnormal dryness of the mouth, blurred vision, slow beating of the heart, and retention of the urine.

Phenylpropanolamine hydrochloride (25 mg per tablet in some cold medicines) and phenylephrine hydrochloride (5 mg per tablet) serve to decrease nasal congestion and dilate the bronchi. These and related drugs, such as epinephrine and amphetamine, are also used in nose drops. It is estimated that one to ten percent of users of such nose drops have reactions from overdosage, such as chronic nasal congestion or personality changes with a psychic craving to continue the use of the drug. Fatalities are rare. The estimated fatal dose for children ranges from 10 mg for epinephrine to 200 mg for phenylpropanolamine.

The prescriptions of physicians for treating colds and other respiratory ailments contain these drugs and other drugs that are equally toxic or more toxic and have a similar incidence of side reactions.

Instead of the warning

KEEP THIS MEDICINE OUT OF REACH OF CHILDREN!

carried by cold medicines, I think that they should say

KEEP THIS MEDICINE OUT OF REACH OF EVERYBODY!
USE ASCORBIC ACID INSTEAD!

The people of the United States spend about $500,000,000 per year on cold medicines. These medicines do not prevent the colds. They may decrease somewhat the misery of the cold, but they also do harm, because of their toxicity and their side effects.

The natural, essential food ascorbic acid, taken in the right amounts at the right time, would prevent most of these colds from developing and would in most cases greatly decrease the intensity of the symptoms in those that do develop. Ascorbic acid is nontoxic, whereas all the cold drugs are toxic, and some of them cause severe side reactions in many people. In every respect, ascorbic acid is to be preferred to the dangerous and only partially effective analgesics, antipyretics, antihistamines, antitussives, bronchodilators, antispasmodics, and central-nervous-system depressants that constitute most medicines sold for relief of the common cold.

CHAPTER 10

How to Control the Common Cold

The following recommendations about intake of ascorbic acid are based upon the evidence and arguments presented in the earlier chapters of this book, including especially those in the publications of Dr. Irwin Stone and Dr. Edmé Régnier, as well as my own observations.

Professor Roger J. Williams and Dr. Gary Deason have concluded that there is a twenty-fold range in the needs of individual guinea pigs for ascorbic acid, and that the range of needs of individual human beings is probably not smaller (Chapter 8). These recommendations include recognition of this biochemical individuality.

First, for good health I recommend the regular ingestion of an adequate amount of ascorbic acid. I estimate that for many people 1 g to 2 g per day (1000 mg to 2000 mg per day) is approximately the optimum rate of ingestion. There is evidence that some people remain in very good health, including freedom from the common cold, year after year through the ingestion of only 250 mg of ascorbic acid per day. The requirements of a few people for ascorbic acid may be expected to be even smaller. For some people optimum health may require larger amounts, up to 5 g per day or more.

The level of ascorbic acid in the blood reaches a maximum in 2 or 3 hours after the ingestion of a moderate quantity, and then gradually decreases, as the ascorbic acid is eliminated in the urine. It may be estimated that 1 g of ascorbic acid taken in four parts during the day (250 mg at breakfast, lunch, dinner, and in the evening) is as effective as 2 g or 3 g taken at one time. Convenience may, however, justify the ingestion of the daily ascorbic acid at one time; for example, at breakfast. It is unlikely that there is any serious consequence of taking it in a single dose. The resistance to infection may well be determined by the lowest concentration in the blood and tissues, however, rather than the average concentration, so that regular ingestion is desirable.

A large quantity of ascorbic acid has a laxative action, especially when it is taken without food. It is probably desirable to take your ascorbic acid at the end of a meal, rather than before the meal.

Since human beings show biochemical individuality, there is the possibility that a person may respond in an unusual way to an increased intake of ascorbic acid. Because ascorbic acid is required as an essential nutrient, and all of our ancestors tolerated it for millions of years, it is very unlikely that anyone would have a serious allergic response to it. There is, however, a slight possibility of allergy to the filler, if tablets are taken. It is, of course, wise to increase or decrease the daily intake of this nutrient gradually.

A few months of experience should be enough to tell you whether the amount of ascorbic acid that you are ingesting approximates the desirable amount, the amount that provides protection against the common cold. If you are taking 1 g per day, and find that you have developed two or three colds during the winter season, it would be wise to try taking a larger daily quantity.

Also, if you are exposed to a cold, by having been in contact with a person suffering from a cold, or if you have become chilled by exposure or tired by overwork or lack of sleep, it would be wise to increase the amount of ascorbic acid ingested.

A convenient way of taking ascorbic acid is to stir the quantity desired, as fine crystals, in a glass of orange juice, where it quickly dissolves. One level teaspoonful is approximately 4 g (more accurately, 4.4 g), so that 1 g is obtained by taking one-quarter of a level teaspoonful of the crystals. The crystals may also be dissolved in tomato juice or cranberry juice, or simply in water, with sugar added if the acid taste is unpleasant. Tablets of ascorbic acid may, of course, be used.

The availability of ascorbic acid as fine crystals and as tablets is discussed in Appendix I.

How to Ameliorate a Cold

The regular use of ascorbic acid in the optimum daily amount appropriate to you as an individual human being may suffice to keep you from catching the common cold or influenza or other infection under most circumstances. But even if, under unusual circumstances, a cold begins to develop, there is still the possibility of ameliorating it by the use of ascorbic acid.

It is wise to carry some 500-mg tablets of ascorbic acid with you at all times. At the first sign that a cold is developing, the first feeling of scratchiness of the throat, or presence of mucus in the nose, or muscle pain or general malaise, begin the treatment by swallowing one or two 500-mg tablets. Continue the treatment for several hours by taking an additional tablet or two tablets every hour.

If the symptoms disappear quickly after the first or second dose of ascorbic acid, you may feel safe in returning to your usual regimen. If, however, the symptoms are present on the second day, the regimen should be continued, with the ingestion of 4 g to 10 g of ascorbic acid per day.

Dr. Regnier has pointed out (1968) that his observations indicate that when a cold is suppressed or averted by the use of an adequate amount of ascorbic acid the viral infection does not disappear at once, but remains suppressed, and that it is accordingly important that the vitamin-C regimen be continued for an adequate period of time. He recommends ingestion of about 4 g of ascorbic acid, in divided doses, per day for the first three or four days, dropping then to about 3 g for three or four days, then to 2 g per day, and then to 1 g per day.

It is not unreasonable that, because of individual variability, the suppression of the disagreeable manifestations of the common cold could be suppressed for some people by a regimen involving the daily ingestion for a few days of a smaller amount of ascorbic acid, 1 g or 2 g per day, and that a larger amount, 10 g or 15 g per day, would be necessary for others.

Ascorbic acid is inexpensive and harmless, even when it is ingested in large amounts. A common cold, when it develops, may involve serious discomfort and suffering, inconvenience and reduced efficiency, and even disability for some days. Moreover, it may lead to the complications of more serious infections. It is accordingly better to overestimate the amount of ascorbic acid needed to control the cold than to underestimate it. A person with a chronic ailment should, of course, consult his physician about his ascorbic-acid intake.

The amount 1 g to 5 g per day of ascorbic acid is not large, compared with the amounts of other foods ingested daily. The recommended daily intake of protein by an adult is 50 g to 70 g or more, corresponding to between 1 and 8 g of each of the eight essential amino acids. Carbohydrates and fats are required for energy. The average amount of carbohydrate ingested by an adult is about 300 g per day, and the average amount of fat is about 100 g per day.

It is recommended by responsible medical authorities that physicians not prescribe antibiotics, such as penicillin, for the common cold. Moreover, there is an additional hazard associated with the injection of an antibiotic, such as penicillin, that can be administered by mouth. Part of the additional hazard is that injections, if carried out with insufficient care, may introduce viruses that can cause diseases into the body. A somewhat larger dose of an antibiotic taken by mouth is often as effective as a dose given by injection.

You must not be disappointed if your physician at first expresses opposition to your use of ascorbic acid as recommended in this book. In the past the medical student has been taught little about vitamins and nutrition in medical school. Fortunately, physicians are now beginning to recognize the value of the vitamins and of orthomolecular therapy in general.

Ascorbic acid can be purchased retail, as fine crystals in 1-kg bottles, for about $10 per kilogram, at the present time (1970). Five hundred grams per year is the amount needed for the regimen described above as one that will avert or greatly ameliorate essentially all colds for many people. At $10 per kilogram, the cost of this regimen comes to $5 per year, as compared with $75 per year estimated in Chapter 1 as the value that might be placed on being essentially free of colds during the year.

If the use of ascorbic acid, as recommended above, were to become general, the price of ascorbic acid would decrease, so that the cost of a year's supply would probably drop as low as one dollar per person. The sum required to protect nearly all the American people against the common cold, two hundred million dollars per year, would then be far less than the amounts now being spent for aspirin and other drugs that are used in the effort to decrease somewhat the severity of the infections, and less than 2 percent of the estimate of fifteen billion dollars made in Chapter 1 as representing the monetary damage done by colds in the United States.

For many years I have analyzed the problem of human suffering and its causes, especially in relation to the role of science in improving human welfare. Despite the recent progress in science and medicine generally, the common cold continues to cause a tremendous amount of suffering. I believe that the application of a simple form of orthomolecular medicine, the use of ascorbic acid, can be effective in averting and ameliorating the common cold, and thus in decreasing the amount of human suffering; and I hope that this book will contribute to achieving this result.

How to Buy Vitamin C

There is only one vitamin C. It is the substance L-ascorbic acid, which is also called ascorbic acid. Sometimes L-ascorbic acid is called natural ascorbic acid, the form that occurs in nature (in foodstuffs), to distinguish it from D-ascorbic acid, a closely related substance that does not have vitamin-C activity. You do not need to worry about whether you are buying vitamin C when you buy ascorbic acid, U.S.P. (United States Pharmacopeia); the inactive form is not on the market.

So-called synthetic ascorbic acid is natural ascorbic acid, identical with the vitamin C in oranges and other foods.

There is no advantage whatever to buying "All-natural Vitamin C," "Wild Rose Hip Super Vitamin C," "Acerola Berries Vitamin C," or similar preparations. In fact, there is the disadvantage that you would waste your money if you bought them, rather than the ordinary ascorbic acid.

The best buy is the pure crystalline substance, in bottles containing 1 kilogram (1000 g, about 2.2 pounds), labelled "Ascorbic Acid, U.S.P., Fine Crystals," or "Ascorbic Acid, U.S.P., Powder."

The manager of the drug departments of one of the large supermarket chains has written me that these drug departments will sell 1-kg bottles of ascorbic acid retail on special order for about $10.50 per bottle ($10.50 per kilogram), and that the price will be lowered if a demand develops.

In connection with our research program, I have bought 100 bottles for $520; that is, $5.20 per 1-kg bottle. With a 40-percent increase for retail sale, this corresponds to a retail price of $7.28 for a 1-kg bottle. I predict that within one year ascorbic acid will be on the shelves of large food stores and drug stores in 1-kg bottles with a retail price of $7.50, and within two or three years with a retail price of $5.00.

It is often convenient to have ascorbic acid available in tablets. Tablets cost more than the pure substance because of the operation of making the tablets. The big tablets (500 mg) are a better buy than small tablets, and they have the advantage of not containing so much filler. I have purchased a bottle of one thousand 500-mg tablets in a discount drug store at a retail price of $7.00, which corresponds to $14.00 per kilogram.

When you buy ascorbic acid, calculate the price per kilogram. If it is more than $20, don't buy, but go to another store. For example, I have before me an advertisement for Rose Hip All Natural Vitamin C tablets, $1.25 for a bottle of 100 tablets. It is stated that three tablets contain 30 mg of ascorbic acid. Hence one tablet contains 10 mg and the bottle of 100 tablets contains 1000 mg, which is 1 gram, at a cost of $1.25. The cost per kilogram is hence $1250, about half the cost of an automobile. This natural-health-products dealer sells vitamin C to his customers at a price about 100 times higher than it should be. The result is that the health of some customers may suffer because they don't have enough money to buy the quantities of vitamins and of good foods that they should be eating.

The dealer also misleads his customers by suggesting that ordinary ascorbic acid is different from "all-natural vitamin C, from organically grown rose hips imported from Northern Europe." The words "organically grown" are essentially meaningless—just part of the jargon used by health-food promoters in making their excess profits, often from elderly people with low incomes. Vitamin C from rose hips is no different from that from any other source, no different from the crystals of ascorbic acid, U.S.P., in a 1-kg bottle.

If you belong to a cooperative market or shop at a large market, ask the manager to order some 1-kg bottles of Ascorbic Acid, U.S.P., fine crystals (or powder), and put them on the shelves for sale. He should be able to get it from the distributor for about $5.00 per 1-kg bottle, wholesale. With the retail increase, the retail price should be between $7.50 and $10.00 for a 1-kg bottle. As mentioned above, tablets cost somewhat more.

Ascorbic acid in the form of fine crystals or crystalline powder kept in a brown bottle is stable indefinitely, and can be kept for years. Dry tablets are also reasonably stable, and can be kept for years in a brown bottle. Solutions of ascorbic acid may be oxidized when exposed to air and light. A solution of ascorbic acid in water may, however, be kept for several days in a refrigerator without significant oxidation. The solubility of ascorbic acid is high; water at ordinary temperatures can dissolve about one third its weight of ascorbic acid.

Everyone should ingest a varied diet, including green vegetables. Such a diet might provide 100 mg to 300 mg of ascorbic acid per day. Most meats contain very little ascorbic acid, less than 5 mg per 100 g (about 4 ounces). Organs such as brains, kidney, and liver, cooked, contain 10 to 30 mg per 100 g. Orange juice contains about 50 mg per 100 g (one glass of fresh juice or freshly reconstituted frozen juice). Green vegetables (properly cooked), such as cabbage, spinach, broccoli, and mustard greens contain 30 to 90 mg per 100 g. Raw black currants and red or green peppers contain 200 to 350 mg per 100 g.

An ordinary good modern diet contains less than the optimum amount of ascorbic acid, because of its inclusion of meat and of processed and cooked foods. Thus for most people it is advisable to include additional ascorbic acid in the diet.

Multivitamin
Food Supplementation

In order to have the best of health, human beings must ingest an adequate quantity of each of the vitamins. The optimum intake no doubt varies from person to person. Probably almost everyone would benefit by supplementing his ordinary foods by the especially important foods called vitamins.

An easy way to carry out this supplementation is by taking a capsule or tablet containing a number of vitamins, a so-called multivitamin preparation. There is only one official multivitamin preparation listed in the United States Pharmacopeia. This preparation is called Decavitamin Capsules or Decavitamin Tablets, U.S.P. Each Decavitamin capsule or tablet (the two have the same composition of active substances) contains ten vitamins in the following amounts:

Vitamin A	4,000 units
Vitamin D	400 units
Ascorbic Acid	75 mg
Thiamine (B_1)	1.0 mg
Riboflavin (B_2)	1.2 mg

Nicotinamide (Niacinamide)	10 mg
Folic Acid	0.25 mg
Pyridoxine (B_6)	2.0 mg
Calcium Pantothenate	5 mg
Cyanocobalamin (B_{12})	0.002 mg

These amounts represent approximately the recommended dietary allowances of the ten vitamins, as given by the Food and Nutrition Board of the National Research Council. These recommended daily dietary allowances, given in the seventh report, 1968, and described as designed for the maintenance of good nutrition of practically all healthy people in the United States, are the following, for a 70-kilogram (154-pound) man:

Vitamin A	5,000 International Units
Vitamin D	400 International Units
Ascorbic Acid	60 mg
Thiamine	1.4 mg
Riboflavin	1.7 mg
Nicotinic Acid	20 mg
(equivalent to the same amount of nicotinamide)	
Folic Acid	0.4 mg
Pyridoxine	2.0 mg
Cyanocobalamin	0.006 mg
Vitamin E	30 International Units

Comparison of these amounts with the amounts in Decavitamin Capsules and Decavitamin Tablets shows that the U.S.P. preparations contain in two capsules or tablets the recommended daily allowance, or somewhat more, for all of the vitamins except B_{12}, cyanocobalamin, for which three tablets would be needed, and vitamin E, which is not included in the Decavitamin Capsules or Tablets.

Multiple vitamins (multivitamins) in capsule or tablet form can be obtained in large drug stores and supermarkets. These food supplements are in packages with the composition given on the package. The composition is usually very nearly the same as the recommended daily dietary allowances, as listed above, except that some of these preparations do not contain folic acid.

The cost of supplementing one's diet with two or three multivitamin capsules or tablets per day is not great. A bottle containing 1000 capsules or 1000 tablets can be purchased from some firms for about $6. (See Burack, *The New Handbook of Prescription Drugs*, 1970.) The cost in large drug stores and supermarkets is about the same; I have bought bottles containing 250 multivitamin tablets for $1.79. Supplementing one's diet by use of these multivitamin preparations accordingly costs only a few dollars per year.

The cost is much greater, five or ten times as much, if the vitamins are obtained with trade names or on prescription. There is no advantage to the preparations with trade names, and no advantage to obtaining the vitamins by prescription.

Moreover, the cost of vitamins is in general considerably higher if they are obtained from special health-product sources. From a representative catalog of such a health-product firm I find that tablets essentially equivalent to Decavitamin Tablets U.S.P. are listed at $15 for 250, which is eight times the price mentioned above.

It is wise not to rely entirely on such a dietary supplement for the essential foods. The essential amino acids are not required as a dietary supplement if an adequate supply of protein is ingested. Moreover, although it is believed that the most important essential nutrients for man are known, there is still the possibility that some have remained undiscovered. For this reason I agree with the specialists in nutrition that everyone should ingest a well-balanced diet, with a good amount of green vegetables, well prepared, and fresh fruits, such as oranges or grapefruit.

If we lived entirely on raw, fresh plant foods, as our ancestors did some millions of years ago, there would be no need for concern about getting adequate amounts of the essential foods, such as the vitamins. The vitamin content of foods is decreased by modern methods of processing and also by cooking. Accordingly it is often necessary to supplement the diet by ingesting additional amounts of these important foods, especially of ascorbic acid, for the reasons discussed earlier in this book.

There is some question whether the so-called bioflavonoids (vitamin P), which are substances extracted from the citrus fruits and other fruits, have any value in supplementing the protective power of ascorbic acid against the common cold. The bioflavonoids are effective in preventing fragility and permeability of the capillaries in guinea pigs, and have been used to some extent to decrease capillary fragility and permeability in humans. Vitamin P has not been included in a recent authoritative treatise, *Vitamins and Coenzymes*, by Wagner and Folkers, 1964. In the study by Franz, Sands, and Heyl (1956), in which it was found that subjects receiving ascorbic acid showed a more rapid improvement in their colds than those not receiving it, no difference was found between those receiving bioflavonoids, either with or without ascorbic acid, and those who did not receive bioflavonoids. Also, as mentioned in Chapter 5, Dr. Régnier (1968) reported that he began his studies by using both ascorbic acid and bioflavonoids, but soon observed that ascorbic acid alone was just as effective as the same amount of ascorbic acid with bioflavonoids.

I conclude that it is likely that bioflavonoids do not have any value, or have very little value, in assisting in the control of the common cold, and accordingly need not be included in the regimen.

Good general nutrition, in addition to an adequate intake of ascorbic acid, is needed for protection against colds and other infections. It has been reported that the susceptibility to colds is decreased by an increase in the daily allowance of vitamin A for some people and of vitamin E for others. It is, however, ascorbic acid for which the ratio between the optimum intake and the usually recommended intake is the greatest and which is shown by the evidence to be the most important food for preventing colds.

Other Studies of Ascorbic Acid and the Common Cold

In the editorial on ascorbic acid and the common cold that was published in *Nutrition Reviews* in 1967 mention is made of ten investigations. Two of them have been described in Chapter 5 (Glazebrook and Thomson, 1942; Ritzel, 1961). The other eight are included among those discussed below.

Tebrock, Arminio, and Johnston reported in 1956 that they had tested the value of ascorbic acid, with or without bioflavonoids, in shortening the period of illness with the common cold. The amount of ascorbic acid administered was very small—only 200 mg per day for three days, beginning when the patient reported that he had a cold. Nearly 2000 patients were studied, with half of them receiving ascorbic acid (total amount 0.6 g) and the other half receiving a placebo or a bioflavonoid capsule. No difference in the duration of the colds was observed. The amount of ascorbic acid used was very much smaller than the amount recommended in this book, in fact, no more than 5 percent of my recommendation.

Bartley, Krebs, and O'Brien (1953) are quoted in the *Nutrition Reviews* editorial as having found that the mean length of colds in subjects deprived of ascorbic acid was twice as great (6.4 days) as for subjects not deprived (3.3 days). Fletcher and Fletcher (1951) stated that supplements of 50 mg to 100 mg of ascorbic acid per day increased the resistance of children to infection. Some value of small amounts of ascorbic acid was reported also by Barnes (1961), Macon (1956), and Banks (1965, 1968). Marckwell (1947) stated that there was a 50-percent chance of stopping a cold if enough ascorbic acid were taken: 0.75 g at once, followed by 0.5 g every three or four hours, continuing on later days if needed.

Bessel-Lorck reported in 1959 that she had given 1 g of ascorbic acid per day to 26 of 46 students in a ski camp in the mountains. After nine days one of the 26 recipients of ascorbic acid and 9 of the 20 controls had developed colds. The patients were treated with 2 g per day, and the 11 remaining controls began to receive 1 g per day. Three of them (and none of the original recipients) developed colds within the next three days. These observations indicate that the ingestion of 1 g of ascorbic acid per day may lead in a few days to the development of significant resistance to infection. This conclusion is statistically significant; the probability that the observations would be made in a uniform population is only 0.3 percent. Accordingly, this work also supports the recommended regimen.

On the other hand, even nearly 3 g per day may not be effective if the treatment is delayed until after the cold has begun. Cowan and Diehl (1950), who with Baker (1942) had found a decrease by 15 percent in the incidence of colds in students regularly taking 200 mg per day, reported no therapeutic effect when the ingestion of ascorbic acid was delayed until the cold was begun and was continued for only three days (2.66 g the first and second days. 1.33 g the third day). A similar lack of effectiveness of 3 g per day, starting after the cold had developed, was also reported by a group of 78 British physicians (Abbott and others, 1968).

Nearly half of the *Nutrition Reviews* editorial is devoted to the 1967 paper by Walker, Bynoe, and Tyrrell, of the Common Cold Research Unit, in Salisbury, England, where the common cold has been studied since 1946. These investigators reported observations on tissue cultures, mice, and human volunteers, and concluded that "there is no evidence that the administration of ascorbic acid has any value in the prevention or treatment of colds produced by five known viruses." Of the 91 human volunteers, 47 received 3 g of ascorbic acid per day for nine days and 44 received a placebo. They were all inoculated with cold viruses (rhinoviruses, influenza B virus, or B814 virus) on the third day. In each of the two groups (47 in the ascorbic-acid group, 44 in the control group), 18 developed colds. There was no significant difference in the severity and duration of the colds.

The number of subjects, 91 in the two groups, was not great enough to permit a statistically significant test of a difference as large as 30 percent in the incidence of colds in the two groups to be made, although a difference of 40 percent, if it had been observed, would have been reported as statistically significant (probability of observation in a uniform population equal to 5 percent). The incidence of colds observed in the subjects receiving ascorbic acid (18/47) was 6 percent less than that in the control group (18/44). This difference is not statistically significant, and the observation does not rule out the possibility of a considerably larger protective effect. Also, this observation does not prove that somewhat larger amounts would not be effective. Both Dr. Stone and Dr. Régnier recommend larger amounts, 4 to 10 g per day. Moreover, these subjects, in England, may have been more depleted of ascorbic acid than those of Dr. Stone and Dr. Régnier, in the United States. The British authorities recommend only one third the daily allowance of ascorbic acid recommended by the U.S. Food and Nutrition Board, and the available food might well have been deficient in this vitamin. The investigators mention that their study was carried out at the time of year (January to May) when the dietary intake of ascorbic acid was expected to be low. This is also the time when a larger intake of ascorbic acid would be needed to achieve the protective level.

There is, of course, the possibility that the inoculations introduced so many virus particles that every inoculated person (33 percent for rhinoviruses, 50 percent for influenza B and B814) who had not developed a specific immunity during the preceding few months would become ill. It is clear that the balance between protection and non-protection by ascorbic acid is a delicate one: 4 g may protect, and 3 g fail to protect; 1 g taken at once when the first sniffle is noticed may protect, 1 g two hours later may fail to protect.

Walker, Bynoe, and Tyrrell begin their report by stating that ascorbic acid is widely used as a prophylactic and therapeutic agent against the common cold. They then write that "though many people use this treatment on themselves and believe it is effective, it is impossible to assess its efficacy."

I do not believe that it is impossible to assess its efficacy. I hope that these investigators, with their extensive experience, will carry out a thorough study, involving placing subjects (with suitable controls) on a regimen of 1 g to 5 g of ascorbic acid per day for months, and another (or combined) study involving ingestion of 1 g or 2 g per hour as soon as symptoms of a cold manifest themselves. The common cold is so great a scourge that the Walker-Bynoe-Tyrrell "Trial of Ascorbic Acid" should be carried through to completion. I hope also that the U.S. National Institutes of Health and other agencies will carry out thorough and reliable studies.

Many other reports on ascorbic acid and the common cold have been published. Some of them are mentioned in a recent book by Dr. Fred R. Klenner (1969). In his medical practice in North Carolina Dr. Klenner has made use of ascorbic acid in amounts 1 g to 20 g per day in treating patients with various viral and bacterial infections. For the common cold he recommends 1.5 g of ascorbic acid taken with fruit juice every hour for ten hours, and continuing at the rate 1 g per hour on the second day. This regimen is nearly the same as that recommended by Dr. Irwin Stone (Chapter 5).

I have examined many other published reports on ascorbic acid and the common cold. I think that those cited above and in Chapter 5 are the most important ones.

Possible Governmental Restriction of the Sale of Ascorbic Acid

There is at the present time (1970) a serious danger that the availability of the important food ascorbic acid will be greatly restricted by action of the United States Government.

Some proposed changes in the regulations about the sale and labeling of dietary supplements, including ascorbic acid, and of foods fortified with vitamins and minerals were announced by James L. Goddard, Commissioner of Foods and Drugs of the U.S. Department of Health, Education, and Welfare, on 9 December 1966 (published in the *Federal Register* for 14 December 1966, 31, 15730). Public hearings on the proposal have been held. There is the possibility that the proposed regulations will go into effect, and that for many people it may become impossible to obtain a supply of vitamins sufficient to keep them in the best of health.

One of the proposals is that vitamins could not be sold to the public (without a physician's prescription) except in tablets or capsules containing not more than certain maximum amounts, approximately equal to the daily allowances recommended by the Food and Nutrition Board of the U.S. National

Research Council. For ascorbic acid (vitamin C) the proposed maximum amount per tablet or capsule that could be sold is 100 mg (even this amount would be restrictively labeled "for pregnant or lactating woman").

The regular intake that I recommend (following Dr. Irwin Stone and my own experience) is 3 g per day, for many people. To obtain this intake I would have to swallow 30 tablets every day. To stop a cold by taking 10 g per day I would have to swallow 100 tablets per day. I think that I would have as much trouble swallowing all of these tablets as I have in swallowing some of the statement made by the Food and Drug Administration in proposing these regulations.

The 100-mg ascorbic acid tablets consist largely of "inert" filler. The large amount of this unwanted substance in 30 or 100 tablets might have some deleterious effect. Also, the 100-mg tablets are expensive—two or three times as expensive (per gram of ascorbic acid) as 500-mg tablets, six or eight times as expensive as ascorbic acid crystals.

The proposal contains the requirement that each package of vitamins should have the following statement in prominent type on the label:

> Vitamins and minerals are supplied in abundant amounts by commonly available foods. Except for persons with special medical needs, there is no scientific basis for recommending routine use of dietary supplements.

This statement is not true. In this book, *Vitamin C and the Common Cold,* I have presented the scientific basis for recommending an increased rate of ingestion of ascorbic acid. Many people, especially children and older people, would have improved health through supplementing their diet with other vitamins also.

It is also proposed to forbid in the labeling, promotional material, or advertising any statement, vignette, or other printed or graphic matter that represents, suggests, or implies

> that a dietary deficiency or threatened dietary deficiency of vitamins and/or minerals is or may be due to loss of nutritive value of food by reason of the soil on which the food is grown, or the storage, transportation, processing, and cooking of food.

. Why should our government forbid anyone to learn or to tell the truth about foods? Why should it be illegal to quote such information as the statement in the handbook *Metabolism* (Altman and Dittmer, 1968) that after storage for three months potatoes contain only half as much ascorbic acid as when fresh? What crime does one commit in quoting the paper of Glazebrook and Thomson (1942), who found that a ration of potatoes (12 ounces) containing 50 mg of ascorbic acid when raw contained only 4 mg, less than one tenth as much, when cooked and reheated for serving?

It is well known that the vitamins in foods are in part destroyed by the storage, transportation, processing, and cooking of the foods. Why should it be forbidden to tell the truth about the dangers of malnutrition and the possibilities of vitamin or mineral deficiencies in foods?

If the Food and Drug Administration wants to help the people, I suggest that it carry on a campaign of education about nutrition and health, including the prices of important foods such as vitamins. It should be pointed out that the "reputable" drug houses market brand-name vitamins that are sold (often on prescription) at prices ten times as high as the equivalent supermarket multivitamin tablets (see Appendix II), and that health-food stores and mail-order houses use outright misrepresentation (such as stating or implying that their own special brands of vitamin C are different from and better than ordinary vitamin C, ascorbic acid) to sell their products to the ignorant and trusting consumer at as much as a hundred times the proper price.

Purchasers of vitamins should learn to read the labels, calculate the cost for a fixed amount of ascorbic acid or other vitamin, and then spend their money carefully.

It is also proposed that it be made illegal to make the following statement:

> That significant segments of the population of the United States are suffering or are in danger of suffering from a dietary deficiency of vitamins or minerals.

But this statement is *true*. One third of the people of the United States are poverty stricken and poorly nourished. They are suffering from a dietary deficiency not only of vitamins and minerals but also of proteins, fats, and carbohydrates. What these malnourished Americans need is money to buy food, and good, sensible advice about nutrition, including the role of the vitamins and minerals.

Many of the more affluent Americans also are suffering from a dietary deficiency. A specialist in nutrition once chided me for writing that many Americans would have improved mental health if they ingested more vitamins; he said that most Americans have enough money to buy food that provides their vitamin requirements. I replied that affluent people might have enough money to buy this good high-vitamin food, and still they might fail to spend it in this way. Cola drinks, potato chips, and hamburgers do not constitute a good diet.

I hope that both the Food and Drug Administration of the Department of Health, Education, and Welfare and the Food and Nutrition Board of the National Research Council will examine the evidence about the optimal daily intake of vitamins, especially ascorbic acid.

I recommend that the Food and Drug Administration give up its attempt to restrict the sale of vitamins, and instead carry out an educational program about how to keep healthy and at the same time avoid being grossly overcharged. And perhaps the Food and Drug Administration will take action against the purveyors of the cold "remedies" mentioned in Chapter 9, and will require that there be on each bottle of aspirin the statement that aspirin is a poison, with fatal dose 0.4 to 0.5 g per kilogram body weight. A similar statement might be required on all the other cold medicines, most of which are more poisonous than aspirin. The suggestion might be included that the safe substance ascorbic acid be used instead of such "remedies."

I am convinced that the value of ascorbic acid in providing protection against infectious disease should now be recognized.

References

Abbott, P., and 77 others (1968), Ineffectiveness of Vitamin C in Treating Coryza, *The Practitioner* 200, 442.

Adams, J. M. (1967), *Viruses and Colds: the Modern Plague*, American Elsevier Publishing Company, New York.

Altman, P. L., and Dittmer, D. S. (1968), *Metabolism*, Federation of American Societies for Experimental Biology, Bethesda, Md.

Andrewes, C. (1965), *The Common Cold*, W. W. Norton & Company, New York.

Anonymous (1967), Ascorbic Acid and the Common Cold, *Nutrition Reviews* 25, 228.

Anonymous (1969), C, the Vitamin with Mystique, *Mademoiselle*, November, p. 189.

Baetgen, D. (1961), Results of Treating Epidemic Hepatitis in Children with High Doses of Ascorbic Acid, *Medizinische Monatsschrift* 15, 30.

Banks, H. S. (1965), Common Cold: Controlled Trials, *Lancet* 2, 790.

Banks, H. S. (1968), Controlled Trials in the Early Antibiotic Treatment of Colds, *The Medical Officer* 119, 7.

Barnes, F. E., Jr. (1961), Vitamin Supplements and the Incidence of Colds in High School Basketball Players, *North Carolina Medical Journal* 22, 22.

Bartley, W., Krebs, H. A., and O'Brien, J. R. P. (1953), *Medical Research Council Special Report Series* No. 280, Her Majesty's Stationery Office, London.

Beadle, G. W., and Tatum, E. L. (1941), Genetic Control of Biochemical Reactions in Neurospora, *Proceedings of the National Academy of Sciences U.S.* 27, 499.

Bessel-Lorck, C. (1959), Prophylaxis against Colds for Youths in a Ski Camp, *Medizinische Welt* 44, 2126.

Bourne, G. H. (1946), The Effect of Vitamin C on the Healing of Wounds, *Proceedings of the Nutrition Society* 4, 204.

Bourne, G. H. (1949), Vitamin C and Immunity, *British Journal of Nutrition* 2, 346.

Burack, R. (1970), *The New Handbook of Prescription Drugs, Official Names, Prices, and Sources for Patient and Doctor*, Pantheon Books, New York.

Burns, J. J., Mosbach, E. H. and Schulenberg, S. (1954), Ascorbic Acid Synthesis in Normal and Drug-treated Rats, *Journal of Biological Chemistry* 207, 679.

Chaudhuri, C. R., and Chatterjee, I. B. (1969), L-Ascorbic Acid, Synthesis in Birds: Phylogenetic Trend, *Science* 164, 435.

Cochrane, W. A. (1965), Overnutrition in Prenatal and Neonatal Life: A Problem?, *Journal of the Canadian Medical Association* 93, 893.

Cowan, D. W., Diehl, H. S., and Baker, A. B. (1942), Vitamins for the Prevention of Colds, *Journal of the American Medical Association* 120, 1267.

Cowan, D. W., and Diehl, H. S., (1950), Antihistaminic Agents and Ascorbic Acid in the Early Treatment of the Common Cold, *Journal of the American Medical Association* 143, 421.

Debré, R., and Celers, J. (1970), *Clinical Virology*, W. B. Saunders Company, Philadelphia, London, Toronto.

DeJong, B. P., Robertson, W. van B., and Schafer, I. A. (1968), Failure to Induce Scurvy by Ascorbic Acid Depletion in a Patient with Hurler's Syndrome, *Pediatrics* 42, 889.

Dreisbach, R. H. (1969), *Handbook of Poisoning: Diagnosis and Treatment*, 6th Edition, Lange Medical Publications, Los Altos, California.

Dugal, L. P. (1961), Ascorbic Acid and Acclimatization to Cold in Monkeys, *Annals of the New York Academy of Science* 92, 307.

Fabricant, N. D., and Conklin, G. (1965), *The Dangerous Cold*, The Macmillan Company, New York.

Fletcher, J. M., and Fletcher, I. C. (1951), Vitamin C and the Common Cold, *British Medical Journal* 1, 887.

Food and Nutrition Board, U.S. National Research Council (1968), *Recommended Dietary Allowances*, Seventh revised edition, National Academy of Sciences Pub. 1694, National Academy of Sciences, Washington, D. C.

Franz, W. L., Sands, G. W., and Heyl, H. L. (1956), Blood Ascorbic Acid Level in Bioflavonoid and Ascorbic Acid Therapy of Common Cold, *Journal of the American Medical Association* 162, 1224.

Gildersleeve, Douglas (1967), Why Organized Medicine Sneezes at the Common Cold, *Fact*, July-August, p. 21.

Glazebrook, A. J., and Thomson, S. (1942), The Administration of Vitamin C in a Large Institution and its Effect on General Health and Resistance to Infection, *Journal of Hygiene* 42, 1.

Gray, G. W. (1941), *The Advancing Front of Medicine*, Whittlesey House, New York.

Greenwood, James (1964), Optimum Vitamin C Intake as a Factor in the Preservation of Disc Integrity, *Medical Annals of the District of Columbia* 33, 274.

Herjanic, M., and Moss-Herjanic, B. L. (1967), Ascorbic Acid Test in Psychiatric Patients, *Journal of Schizophrenia* 1, 257.

Hindson, T. C. (1968), Ascorbic Acid for Prickly Heat, *Lancet*, June 22, p. 1347; September 21, p. 681.

Holmes, H. N. (1946), The Use of Vitamin C in Traumatic Shock, *Ohio State Medical Journal* 42, 1261.

Isaacs, A., and Lindenmann, J. (1957), Virus Interference. I. The interferon, *Proceedings of the Royal Society of London*, B147, 258.

Klenner, F. R. (with Bartz, F. H.) (1969), *The Key to Good Health: Vitamin C*, Graphic Arts Research Foundation, Chicago, Ill.

Kodicek, E. H., and Young, F. G. (1969), Captain Cook and Scurvy, *Notes and Records of the Royal Society of London*, 24, 43.

Kogan, B. A. (1970), *Health*, Harcourt, Brace and World, Inc., New York, Chicago, San Francisco, Atlanta.

Kubala, A. L., and Katz, M. M. (1960), Nutritional Factors in Psychological Test Behavior, *Journal of Genetic Psychology* 96, 343.

Macon, W. L. (1956), Citrus Bioflavonoids in the Treatment of the Common Cold, *Industrial Medicine and Surgery* 25, 525.

Marckwell, N. W. (1947), Vitamin C in the Prevention of Colds, *Medical Journal of Australia* 34, 777.

Paul, J. H., and Freese, H. L. (1933), An Epidemiological and Bacteriological Study of the "Common Cold" in an Isolated Arctic Community (Spitsbergen), *American Journal of Hygiene* 17, 517.

Pauling, L. (1968), Orthomolecular Somatic and Psychiatric Medicine, *Journal of Vital Substances and Diseases of Civilization*, 14, 1.

Pauling, L. (1968), Orthomolecular Psychiatry, *Science* 160, 265.

Pauling, L. (1970), Evolution and the Need for Ascorbic Acid, *Proceedings of the National Academy of Sciences U.S.* 64, December issue.

Regnier, E. (1968), The Administration of Large Doses of Ascorbic Acid in the Prevention and Treatment of the Common Cold, Parts I and II, *Review of Allergy* 22, 835, 948.

Ritzel, G. (1961), Ascorbic Acid and Infections of the Respiratory Tract, *Helvetica Medica Acta* 28, 63.

Salomon, L. L., and Stubbs, D. W. (1961), Some Aspects of the Metabolism of Ascorbic Acid in Rats, *Annals of the New York Academy of Sciences* 92, 128.

Schlegel, J. U., Pipkin, G. E., Nishimura, R., and Schultz, G. N. (1970), The Role of Ascorbic Acid in the Prevention of Bladder Tumor Formation, *Journal of Urology* 103, 155.

Sokoloff, B., Hori, M., Saelhof, C. C., Wrzolek, T., and Imai, T. (1966), Aging, Atherosclerosis, and Ascorbic Acid Metabolism, *Journal of the American Geriatric Society* 14, 1239.

Stare, F. J. (1969), *Eating for Good Health*, Cornerstone Library, New York.

Stone, I. (1965), Studies of a Mammalian Enzyme System for Producing Evolutionary Evidence on Man, *American Journal of Physical Anthropology* 23, 83.

Stone, I. (1966a), On the Genetic Etiology of Scurvy, *Acta Geneticae Medicae et Gemellologiae* 15, 345.

Stone, I. (1966b), Hypoascorbemia, the Genetic Disease Causing the Human Requirement for Exogenous Ascorbic Acid, *Perspectives in Biology and Medicine* 10, 133.

Stone, I. (1967), The Genetic Disease Hypoascorbemia, *Acta Geneticae Medicae et Gemellologiae* 16, 52.

Tebrock, H. E., Arminio, J. J., and Johnston, J. H. (1956), Usefulness of Bioflavonoids and Ascorbic Acid in Treatment of Common Cold, *Journal of the American Medical Association* 162, 1227.

Wagner, A. F., and Folkers, K. (1964), *Vitamins and Coenzymes*, Interscience Publishers, New York.

Walker, G. H., Bynoe, M. L., and Tyrrell, D. A. J. (1967), Trial of Ascorbic Acid in Prevention of Colds, *British Medical Journal* 1, 603.

Williams, R. J. (1956), *Biochemical Individuality*, John Wiley and Sons, New York.

Williams, R. J. (1967), *You Are Extraordinary*, Random House, New York.

Williams, R. J., and Deason, G. (1967), Individuality in Vitamin C Needs, *Proceedings of the National Academy of Sciences U.S.* 57, 1638.

Willis, G. C., and Fishman, S. (1955), Ascorbic Acid Content of Human Arterial Tissue, *Canadian Medical Association Journal* 72, 500.

Wilson, C. W. M. (1967), Ascorbic Acid and Colds, *British Medical Journal* 2, 698.

Wilson, C. W. M., and Low, H. S. (1970), Ascorbic Acid and Upper Respiratory Inflammation, *Acta Allergolica* 24, 367.

Wolfer, J. A., Farmer, C. J., Carroll, W. W., and Manshardt, D. O. (1947), An Experimental Study in Wound Healing in Vitamin-C Depleted Human Subjects, *Surgery, Gynecology, and Obstetrics* 84, 1.

Yandell, H. R. (1951), The Treatment of Extensive Burns, *American Surgeon* 17, 351.

Zamenhof, S., and Eichhorn, H. H. (1967), Study of Microbial Evolution through Loss of Biosynthetic Functions: Establishment of "Defective" Mutants, *Nature* 216, 456.

Zuckerkandl, E., and Pauling, L. (1962), Molecular Disease, Evolution, and Genic Heterogeneity, *In* Kasha, M., and Pullman, B., eds., *Horizons in Biochemistry* (Szent-Györgyi Dedicatory Volume), Academic Press, New York, p. 189.

Index

About the Author

Linus Pauling was born in Portland, Oregon, on 28 February 1901. His father was a druggist who died when Linus was nine years old. Linus worked his way through the Oregon Agricultural College in Corvallis, where he majored in chemical engineering. As an undergraduate he showed great promise and helped to support himself by teaching chemistry. Because of his financial responsibility for his mother and two younger sisters, he dropped out of his college studies for one year and worked as a full-time teaching assistant in the quantitative analysis courses. (He first met his future wife, Ava Helen Miller, when she was a student in a chemistry course that he taught.) During the summers he worked at a variety of jobs, mainly as a paving-plant inspector.

After receiving his degree in 1922, he earned his doctorate at the California Institute of Technology in 1925, then went on to eighteen months of study in Munich, Zurich, and Copenhagen. He returned to the California Institute of Technology as a member of the faculty, and he remained there until 1964, when he became Research Professor of the Physical and Biological Sciences in the Center for the Study of Democratic Institutions in Santa Barbara, California. In 1968, after spending two years on the faculty of the University of California, San Diego, he moved to Stanford University, where he is Professor of Chemistry.

Linus Pauling has long been deeply concerned with the alleviation of human suffering, and he has brought his scientific knowledge to bear on such problems as the causes of genetic mutation, the transmission of aberrant genes, and the deleterious effects of protein molecules with abnormal structure. On occasions, his views have led him to take strong public positions—some decidedly unpopular or unpolitic—against cigaret smoking, against the maintenance of preventable hereditary diseases in human populations, against the testing, proliferation and use of atomic and nuclear weapons, and against war in general.

His achievements in science, medicine, and the promotion of human welfare have brought him countless honors, such as the Phillips Medal of the American College of Physicians for his contributions to internal medicine, the Gold Medal of the French Academy of Medicine, the Baxter Award in anesthesiology, the Rudolf Virchow Medal, the Thomas Addis Medal of the American Nephrosis Foundation, the *Modern Medicine* Award, the Humanist of the Year Award, and many others, including dozens of honorary degrees and election to honorary membership in twenty scientific societies in twelve countries. Linus Pauling has been awarded two Nobel Prizes: the 1954 Nobel Prize for Chemistry and the 1962 Nobel Prize for Peace.

His principal research at present is on the molecular basis of disease, including mental disease. He has published more than four hundred papers, most of which present the results of original investigations, and he is the author of a number of influential books, including *Introduction to Quantum Mechanics* (with E. B. Wilson, Jr.), *The Nature of the Chemical Bond*, *General Chemistry*, *College Chemistry*, *The Architecture of Molecules* (with Roger Hayward), and *No More War!*.